AF820975

A Brief Introduction to SARS CoV-2

A Brief Introduction to SARS CoV-2

Md. Takim Sarker

ELIVA PRESS

ISBN: 978-99949-8-019-2

Cover Design: Eliva Press
Cover Image: Freepik Premium
Email: info@elivapress.com
Website: www.elivapress.com

This Eliva Press imprint is published by the registered company Eliva Press Global Ltd. part of Eliva Press S.R.L. Publishing Group

The registered company address is: Pope Hennessy Street Level 2, Hennessy Tower Port Louis, Mauritius
Eliva Press S.R.L. Publishing Group address is: Bulevardul Moscova 21, Chisinau, Moldova, Europe

Title: A brief introduction to SARS CoV-2

ACKNOWLEDGEMENT

All praises are to the almighty, the merciful ruler of the universe who enables me to complete this book. I am very much glad to express my gratitude, sincere appreciation and indebtedness to A. Q. Fuad Hasan for his invaluable assistance and support. Otherwise, it would be very difficult and troublesome to complete this book.

Finally, I am grateful to my family members for their endless support, encouragement and love.

Table of Contents

.... 5

Chapter: 1 5

What is SARS CoV-2? 5

1.1 Background 6

1.2 Invasion of SARS-CoV-2 7

1.3 Origin of SARS-CoV-2 7

1.4 Classification of Coronavirus 8

1.5 Structure of SARS-CoV-2 9

Chapter: 2 11

Life Cycle of SARS-CoV-2 11

2.1 Early Stage 12

2.2 Advanced Stage 14

Chapter: 3 16

Molecular insight into SARS CoV-2 16

3.1 Genome Organization of SARS-CoV-2 17

3.2 Mutation in SARS-CoV-2 19

Chapter: 4 21

Aftermath of the pandemic 21

4.1 Epidemiology of COVID-19 22

4.2 Fatality Rate of the Pandemic 23

Chapter: 5 25

Pathogenesis Process of SARS CoV-2 25

5.1 Transmission 26

5.2 Pathological Process 26

5.3 Host Response 27

Chapter: 6 29

Post-Infection Outcomes 29

6.1 Clinical Features 30

6.2 Disease Prognosis 31

Chapter: 7 33

Diagnostic Strategies for COVID-19 33
Chapter: 8 36
Prevention against COVID-19 36
8.1 Preventive Measures 37
8.2 Treatment 39
8.3 Vaccination 42
8.4 Boosting Immunity 45
Chapter: 9 46
Infection Associated Factors 46
9.1 Gender Biases 47
9.2 Ethnic Differences 47
9.3 Environmental Effect 48
9.4 Blood Group and Coronavirus 49
Chapter: 10 50
Future thoughts on COVID-19 50

Chapter: 1

What is SARS CoV-2?

1.1 Background

In late December 2019, the novel coronavirus strain, severe acute respiratory syndrome (SARS-CoV-2), was first traced at the Wuhan metropolis of China's Hubei province (Hui et al., 2020). Though the virus was limited in China during the very early phase of the coronavirus disease 2019 (COVID-19) outbreak, the current scenario is quite devastating throughout the globe. The ongoing pandemic has not only created a massive burden on the universal health care system but also impacted global human beings' social, economic, and health measures (Hossain, Ahmmed, Rahman, et al., 2021; Hui et al., 2020). The causative agent of this outbreak, a type of ß-coronavirus that emerged from unknown or mysterious sources, is SARS-CoV-2, which belongs to the Coronaviridae family (Cyranoski, 2020). The world health organization (WHO) declared this public health emergency as a pandemic on 11 March 2020 (Hossain, Kuddus, & Rahman, 2021). As of September 2021, the global community has counted around 234 million cases and near 4.8 million deaths from this infectious disease and its imposed complications. However, at the current time more than 210 million SARS-CoV-2 infected patients have recovered from this infection (*Worldometer*, n.d.). As this pathogenic virus has newly emerged, the exact mechanism of pathogenesis and its biochemical pathway are still vague and unclear. The spike protein of SARS-COV-2 might have a strong affinity towards the host cell receptor, enhancing its much higher human-to-human transmission (Yin et al., 2020). The primary investigation has revealed that this viral particle infects the respiratory tract and causes respiratory complications ranging from very simple clinical manifestations of hypoxia to acute respiratory distress syndrome (ARDS) (N. Chen et al., 2020; Leung et al., 2020).

Although both the infection and mortality rates were improving, the most virulent variant, the delta variant, has evolved in most countries of the world and worsened the situation with record-breaking infections (Bari et al., 2021; Hossain, Soma, Islam, et al., 2021). Furthermore, WHO has officially declared the earliest onset of symptoms as having been on 8 December 2019 and set a Public Health Emergency of International Concern (PHEIC) on 1 February 2020 (*Novel Coronavirus – China*, n.d.). There are two opinions towards this pathogen. The first is that the origin of this virus is laboratory-based. The second opinion proffers evidence from genomic information suggesting this virus is unique compared to previous coronaviruses (*Covid-19*, n.d.). The cause of COVID-19's severity is well known, and is because it has s1, s2 polybasic cleavage sites in its spike glycoprotein which lead to high binding affinity with ACE-2 receptors (Nao et al., 2017; Samadizadeh et al., 2021). According to a comparison between SARS-CoV-2, SARS (Severe Acute Respiratory Syndrome), and MERS (Middle East Respiratory syndrome) concerning their appearance in community transmission across the globe, SARS-COV-2 appeared at the top. The SARS-COV-2 has shown the highest projected basic reproductive number (R0) of (2–3.58) whereas the R0 was (1.7–1.9) and <1 for SARS and MERS, respectively (J. T. Wu et al., 2020; P. Wu et al., 2020). However, the aim of this comprehensive study is to give an overview of the virus and its origin, including its classification, structure, life cycle, genomic constitution, mutation, epidemiology, prognosis, and pathogenesis. We also summarize the aftermath of the infection, treatments, disease associated factors, and the methods of prevention as guided by public health experts in different sections of our literature review.

1.2 Invasion of SARS-CoV-2

COVID-19 is an infectious disease caused by the infection of SARS severe acute respiratory syndrome coronavirus 2. Coronavirus (CoV) belongs to the RNA virus families that are organized varyingly in animal species. It can invade the respiratory tract, gastrointestinal systems, and the hepatic and nervous systems in humans (Y. Chen et al., 2020). Underneath the electron microscope, it appears to be a crown-like structure because of spike glycoproteins (Cascella et al., 2022). CoVs cause about 5 to 10% of acute respiratory infections. It is reported that 2% of the global population is regarded as healthy carriers of these viruses (Y. Chen et al., 2020). In immune-competent individuals, these CoVs result in self-limiting respiratory infections and common colds. In the case of aged people and immune-compromised individuals, CoVs can affect the lower respiratory tracts (Cascella et al., 2022). Yet, functional deactivation of these viruses can be attained by using ether (75%), ethanol (60%), and chlorine-containing disinfectants (Hassan et al., 2020).

1.3 Origin of SARS-CoV-2

Like SARS-CoV and MERS, SARS-CoV-2 also displays strong similarities with viruses of bat origin (W. Li et al., 2005). The whole-genome alignment between the SARS-CoV-2 and the strains from Rhinolophus affinis species (Bat-CoV RaTG13) from Yunnan province matched up to 96%. (Z. P et al., 2020). Additionally, it is clearly seen that SARS-CoV-2 and previously occurring

SARS CoV and MERS harbor bats as a common source (Table 1) (Kakodkar et al., 2020, p. 19). In addition, the study suspects pangolins as the natural stockpile of SARS-CoV-2. This claim was based upon the result inferred by aligning the genome contigs among SARS-CoV-2-like coronaviruses such as Pangolin-CoV, previously sampled from the lung tissue of two dead Malayan pangolins (Liu et al., 2019). The overall genome sequence of Pangolin-CoV had a 91.02% similarity with SARS-CoV-2 and a 90.55% similarity with Bat-CoV RaTG13 (Kakodkar et al., 2020; T. Zhang et al., 2020, p. 1).

Table 1. Synopsis of the natural reservoir, median host, and target host for major coronaviruses.

Virus	Source of Virus	Transitional Host	Final Host
SARS-CoV-1 (SARS-2002)	SARS-like Bat-CoV	Civet cat	Human
MERS-CoV (MERS 2012)	SARS-like Bat-CoV	Camel	Human
SARS-CoV-2 (COVID-2019)	Bat-CoV RaTG13	Pangolin (Pangolin-CoV)	Human

1.4 Classification of Coronavirus

SARS-CoV-2 is a large, enveloped, and single-stranded RNA virus that is a member of the Coronaviridae family. The Coronaviridae family can be genotypically and serologically categorized into two subfamilies **(Figure 1)**, such as (1) Coronaviridae that consist of alpha, beta, gamma, and delta coronavirus, and (2) Torovirinae that includes unknown genera of Torovirus (G. Lu et al., 2015). To date, a total of seven types of coronaviruses have been found susceptible to cause infection in humans, including α CoVs (HCoV-NL63 and HCoV-229E) and β CoVs (SARS-CoV, MERS-CoV, HCoV-HKU1, HCoV-OC43, and SARS-CoV-2) (S & J, 2009). Out of these, three (SARS-CoV, MERS-CoV, and SARS-CoV-2) are considered highly deleterious for infecting the lower respiratory tract. In contrast, other species are associated with upper respiratory tract infection with mild symptoms (G. Lu et al., 2015). Gene characterization revealed that bats and rodents are the primal gene root of alpha-CoV and beta-CoV. On the other hand, species that include avians are considered as genetic sources of gamma-CoV and delta-CoV (*WHO, 2020*, n.d.). Genome classification reports of the novel variant have shown an 89% nucleotide identity with bat SARS-like CoV-ZXC21 (Chan, Kok, et al., 2020; Y. Chen et al.,

2020). Concurrently, 82% of matching nucleotides have been found in the human SARS virus (Chan, Kok, et al., 2020).

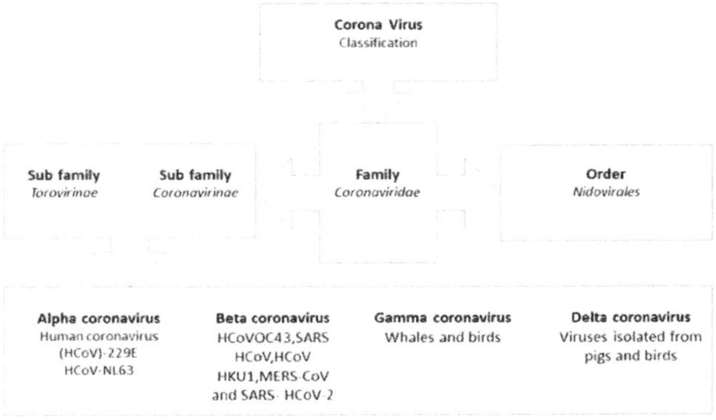

Figure 1. Scientific classification of coronavirus.

1.5 Structure of SARS-CoV-2

SARS-CoV-2 possesses a single and positive-stranded RNA virus enfolded in a lipid bilayer, as shown in (Figure 2) (R. Lu et al., 2020; F. Wu et al., 2020).

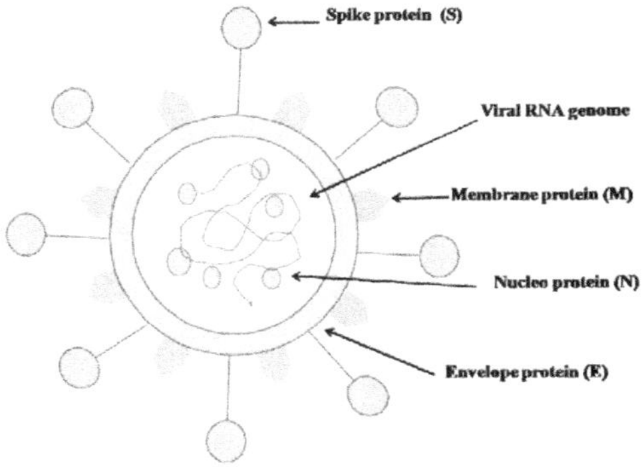

Figure 2. Structural view of SARS-CoV-2.

The lipid bilayer merges into the host's cell membrane, delivering a positive RNA strand into the cytoplasm and seeding the translation of different viral proteins. The newly replicated viral proteins and RNA genome reconcile into new viruses, which eventually rush out of the cell (Qin et al., 2019; Z et al., 2004). SARS-CoV-2 is very weak when susceptible to heat and ultraviolet (Cascella et al., 2022). The spike protein (S-protein) is a glycoprotein expressed as a homotrimer on the viral counterpart, called the viral envelope (F. Li, 2016). Each S-protein is comprised of S1 and S2 subunits. S1 incorporates a receptor-binding domain that spots receptors on the host cells, and S2 modulates the membrane fusion. This viral S-protein ties up with the human ACE2 (Angiotensin Converting Enzyme 2) receptor protein (Nainu et al., 2020). Tissues such as lung, heart, kidney, and adipose are rich with ACE2 receptors (Gupte et al., 2008; Turner et al., 2004).

Chapter: 2

Life Cycle of SARS-CoV-2

The virus particle seems to follow two stages of their complete lifespan: (1) Early stage (entry and initiation, S protein cleavage, membrane fusion) and (2) Advanced stage (translation and RNA replication, virion release) (Figure 3) (Z. P et al., 2020; Poduri et al., 2020, p. 19; Wrapp et al., 2020).

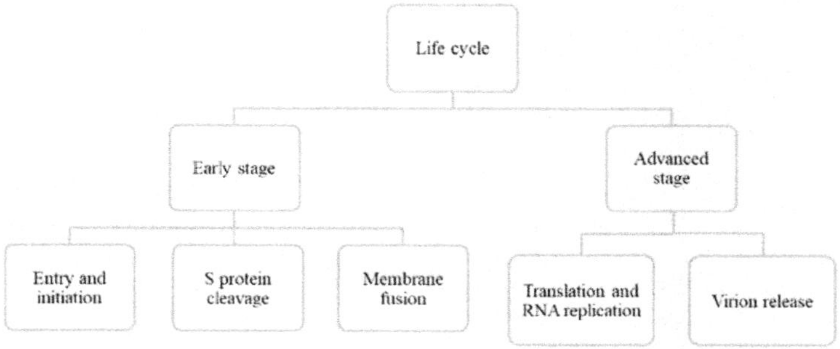

Figure 3. Schematic representation of SARS-CoV-2 entire life cycle.

2.1 Early Stage

2.1.1 Entry and Initiation

All SARS CoVs, MERS, and SARS-CoV-2 possess an S protein that goes through a cleavage event by fusion proteins (Figure 4). An RBD (receptor-binding domain) at the spike protein enables ACE2 (Angiotensin-converting enzyme 2), the host receptor protein, to initiate membrane fusion activity. SARS-CoV-2 shows a higher binding affinity with the ACE2 receptor than any other coronavirus variant, even 20-fold greater than SARS-CoV (Bar-On et al., 2020). ACE2 receptors are located in different parts of our body, including oral mucosa, nasal epithelium, vascular endothelium, lungs, kidney, small intestine, testis, colon, heart, and brain [41,42]. A study conducted by Devaux et al. (Devaux et al., 2020) reported 32 different ACE2 receptors, including seven hotspot variants specified in the different populations. In addition, it is experimentally found that proteases such as cathepsins, human airway trypsin-like proteases, trypsin, furin, and transmembrane protease serine protease (2/4) (TMPRSS) assist in proteolytic cleaving of the S protein into S1/S2 subunits (Belouzard et al., 2009; Gierer et al., 2013; Millet & Whittaker, 2014; Park et al., 2016). The furin protease entry is called endocytosis, whereas TMPRSS (2/4) adopts a direct fusion mechanism (Al-Horani et al., 2020).

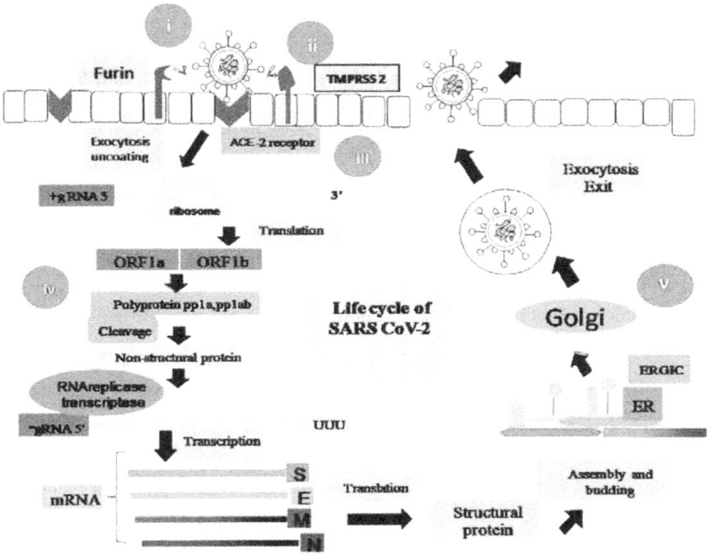

Figure 4. A schematic representation of the entire life cycle of SARS-CoV-2. (i) The entry of the virus particle is initiated by binding of Spike (S) glycoprotein to the ACE2 receptor of the host cell. (ii) The S glycoprotein is cleaved into S1/S2 either by TMPRSS2 or by the furin protease, in association with some cofactors. (iii) S2 stalk domain undergoes a conformational change and facilitates the fusion between the host cell membrane and the virus envelope protein. (iv) In this advanced stage, host cell machinery is used by the virus to translate viral polyprotein pp1a and pp1ab into nsps. The RNA genome and N protein are made in the host cell cytoplasm and the S, E, and M structural proteins are packaged in the endoplasmic reticulum (ER). (v) The mature virion is transferred to the Golgi body followed by exocytosis, budding, or cell death.

2.1.2 S Protein Cleavage

There are two pathways to S protein cleavage. The first is by protease TMPRSS (2/4) in the host cell, and the second is by furin and furin-like proteases (Al-Horani & Kar, 2020). TMPRSS (2/4) belongs to type II transmembrane serine protease found extensively in gastrointestinal, urogenital, and respiratory tracts (Hussain et al., 2020, p. 2). In contrast, the furin and furin-like proteases belong to a group called proprotein convertases, a type I transmembrane protein. It converts the S protein into globular S1 and bio-membrane anchored stalk S2 domain (Brielle et al., 2020). Interestingly there is no compensation activity between TMPRSS (2/4) and furin and furin-like proteases; therefore, halting either of them can be a promising target zone for drug discovery (Khadim Sheikh et al., 2020, p. 2).

2.1.3 Membrane Fusion

There are three mechanisms of membrane fusion. The first is endocytosis, the second is direct fusion, and the third is the proteolytic activity of cathepsins, TMPRSS (2/4), the furin proteases, or other trypsin-like proteases that penetrate through into the endosomes or lysosomes of the cell (Al-Horani & Kar, 2020).

2.2 Advanced Stage

2.2.1 Translation and RNA Replication

The step of replication and transcription occurs after the entry of viral RNA (positive single-stranded) (Hartenian et al., 2020). It involves activities like (1) RNA synthesis, (2) template proofreading, and (3) mRNA capping. The NSPs (non-structural protein) domain initially comprising two polypeptides further generates non-structural proteins like papain-like protease, PLpro (nsp3), main protease, Mpro (nsp5), and RNA-dependent RNA polymerase, RdRp (nsp12). Host proteases are utilized during the processing of the initial two polypeptides. The further processing activity is undergone by the PLpro and Mpro of the virus (Y. Gao et al., 2020b; R. Lu et al., 2020; L. Zhang, Lin, et al., 2020). RdRp plays the focal role in viral replication by the catalysis activity of nsp12, along with nsp7 and nsp8 as cofactors (Y. Gao et al., 2020a). The RNA proofreading and capping of the mRNA are processed by the nsp14. Apart from nsp14, the capping machinery comprises nsp13, nsp16, and nsp10 as cofactors. mRNA capping is inevitable for viral stability and protection against host immunity (Ramanathan et al., 2016; Romano et al., 2020; Shannon et al., 2020; Shereen et al., 2020; Shu et al., 2020). In the host cell cytoplasm, two of the most vital proteins, including N structural protein and the virus RNA, are biosynthesized, and the rest of the structural proteins(S, E, M) are produced in the host's endoplasmic reticulum (ER) (Al-Horani & Kar, 2020).

2.2.2 Virion Packing and Release

The genome is affected by the infection if it occurs within the middle of the ER–Golgi compartment (Al-Horani et al., 2020; Atri et al., 2020; Du et al., 2009; Jiang et al., 2020). The virus may leave the host cell either via exocytosis, budding, or cell death. Most often, undeveloped virion adopts the budding process. At the same time, a mature virus is ejected from the host cell through exocytosis. In some cases, virus particles crack the host cell lysosomes and, in the long run, prompt cell demise. The new virus particles either can contaminate new cells or be delivered into the climate, focusing on another host (Buratta et al., 2020; Malik, 2020).

Chapter: 3

Molecular insight into SARS CoV-2

3.1 Genome Organization of SARS-CoV-2

Human coronaviruses have initially been traced back to the late 1960s, expressing some mild symptoms in the population, similar to the common cold (Kahn & McIntosh, 2005). The date of the first published genomic sequence of SARS-CoV-2 was 24 January 2020, which was an open-access publication. It was found by Wei et al. as a recombinant sequence after the codon usage analysis. However, this notion was disproved by Paraskevis' full-genome evolutionary analysis and Chen's Simplot investigation (Ji et al., 2020; Paraskevis et al., 2020). According to the present study, it is found that SARS-CoV-2 is a new type of positive-sense, single-stranded RNA virus in the Betacoronavirus genus from the Coronaviridae family (L. Chen et al., 2020; R. Lu et al., 2020; Paraskevis et al., 2020). This novel virus' non-segmented whole genome length is 29,891 to 29,903 nucleotides, making it one of the largest viruses among RNA viruses (Cascella et al., 2022). Akin to SARS-CoV and MERS-CoV, the novel SARS-CoV-2 genome carries two untranslated regions (UTRs), 5′-methylated cap and 3′poly-A tail structure, and a single open reading frame (ORF) that codes for a single polyprotein (Chan, Kok, et al., 2020; L. Chen et al., 2020). The 5'-end of the SARS-CoV-2 genome organization is composed of viral replicase (ORF1a and ORF1b)-4 structural proteins (nucleocapsid (N), envelope protein (E), spike protein (S), and membrane protein (M)) and the 3′-end encodes some accessory protein genes, such as ORF 3a, 7, and 8, which are arranged alongside the structural proteins **(Figure 5)** (Chan, Kok, et al., 2020; Chan, Yuan, et al., 2020; L. Chen et al., 2020; R. Lu et al., 2020; Paraskevis et al., 2020; F. Wu et al., 2020).

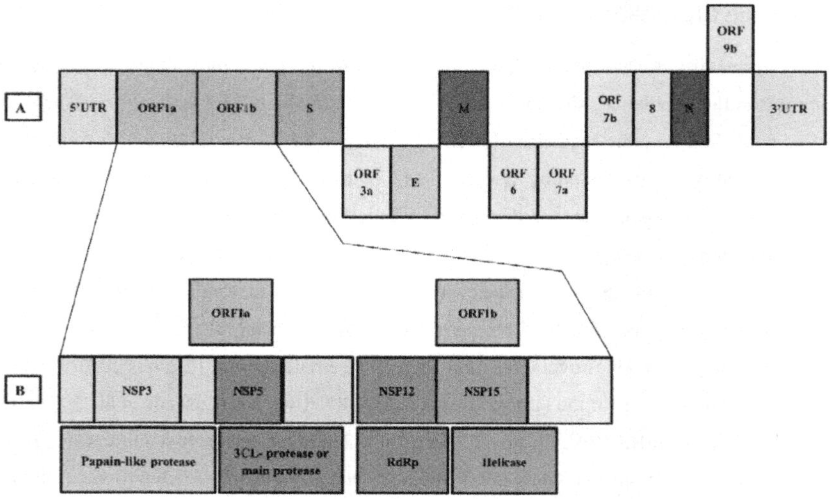

Figure 5. Genome organization of SARS-CoV-2. (A) The whole genome is arranged in the following order; 5′ UTR-ORF1a—ORF1b-Spike protein (S)—ORF 3a—Envelope protein (E)—Membrane protein (M)-ORF 6-ORF 7a—ORF 8—Nucleocapsid (N)—ORF 9b—3′ UTR. (B) Viral replicase proteins (ORF1a and ORF1b) include nsp3 (Papain-like protease), nsp5 (Main proteas), nsp12 (RNA dependent RNA polymerase), and nsp13 (Helicase).

In the SARS-CoV-2 genome, the ORF1a and ORF1b cover about 66% of the entire genome, encoding 16 non-primary proteins (nsps), whereas the remaining 33% encodes adornment proteins and underlying proteins (L. Chen et al., 2020; Hossain, Soma, Islam, et al., 2021). The source of tests was gathered from bronchoalveolar lavage liquid or throat swabs, the Huanan fish market, and lung injuries of patients contributed as an intermediary host in virus transmission (Liu et al., 2019). In recent times, sequences from diverse regions have been recorded in various public databases, making virus tracking a lot more feasible than previously (Hadfield et al., 2018).. A phylogenetic report showed about a 96.2% arrangement comparability among Bat-CoV and SARS-CoV-2 genomes. Genomic grouping character information likewise showed 79.0% and

50.0% succession similarity with SARS-CoV and MERS-CoV, respectively (Ge et al., 2020, p. 19). Surprisingly, genomic comparison from a dead Malayan Pangolin (Manis javanica) with SARS-CoV-2 matched up to 91.02%, indicating that Pangolin could have

3.2 Mutation in SARS-CoV-2

SARS-CoV-2 displays very little sequence diversity due to having a proofreading mechanism, yet there are still chances for natural selection to occur in its favor (Benvenuto et al., 2020)(Fauver et al., 2020; Sevajol et al., 2014; Smith et al., 2013). The more SARS-CoV-2 pandemic remains in the population, the greater its possibility to gather immunologically associated mutations, even after the vaccine is available (Chibo & Birch, n.d.; Y. Guan et al., 2003; Ren et al., 2015; Song et al., 2005; Vijgen et al., 2005). Scientists are solely focused on understanding the evolutionary mechanisms of SARS-CoV-2, including mutation, recombination, and tracing for indels in the genome as they were found in previously discovered coronaviruses (Benvenuto, Giovanetti, et al., 2020). Experiments with the evidence of antigenic drift were seen in previous strains, such as OC43, 229E, and SARS CoV-1, but have not yet been found in SARS-CoV-2 (Chibo & Birch, n.d.; Cohen, 2020; Y. Guan et al., 2003; Ren et al., 2015; Song et al., 2005; Vijgen et al., 2005; Yu et al., 2020). In 2003/2004 viruses, the point mutation D480A/G on the receptor binding domain (RBD) spread with an impactful prevalence in humans and civet cats. In vitro, recapitulated elevation of D480A/G was induced due to immune pressure by neutralizing antibody 80R (Sui et al., 2008). Likewise, point mutations were detected to be worthwhile as an inhibitor for neutralizing antibodies in SARS-CoV-1 and MERS-CoV (Sui et al., 2008; X.-C. Tang et al., 2014). An evolutionary analysis on 351 sequences found two mutations in nsp6 and near the ORF10 region in earlier COVID-19 strains may confer less stability to protein structures. Notably, the nsp6 creates autophagosomes and is available in the endoplasmic reticulum (ER) of both alpha and beta coronaviruses. Accordingly, the mutation in nsp6 may confer a noteworthy change in the expression of SARS-CoV to its host, especially in the autophagic lysosomal system (Benvenuto, Angeletti, et al., 2020). In SARS-CoV-2, another significant amino acid change, D614G, has been traced to appear recurrently in the spike protein worldwide. Before the G614 variant, the original D614 form was firmly retained. An A-to-G mutation gave rise to D614G substitution in the Wuhan reference strain at positions 23,403 (Korber et al., 2020, p.). In early March of 2019, G614 was infrequent worldwide, but gradually thriving in Europe. Eventually, variants carrying the D614G substitution were designated as "G clade". Three additional mutations are also found to be present concurrently with the D614G variant, namely: (1) a C-to-T mutation at position 241, according to Wuhan reference sequence in the 5′ UTR, (2) a C-to-T silent mutation at position 3037, and (3) a C-to-T mutation at position 14,408 (RdRp P323L). Currently, the haplotype containing these four interlinked mutations is starting to be found frequently in Europe, continuing to North America, Oceania, and finally Asia. A study found evidence of higher titers (elevated 2.6–9.3 times) for the G614 variant in infected patients' samples with lower Ct (cycle threshold) value in vivo, indicating higher viral load; yet, this does not confirm disease severity (J. T. Wu et al., 2020). However, G614 may induce spike stability and membrane fusion (L. Zhang, Jackson, et al., 2020).

Chapter: 4

Aftermath of the pandemic

4.1 Epidemiology of COVID-19

A few measures are regularly used to decide the death pace of a pestilence flare-up (*CDC,2021*, n.d.). Regular epidemiological terms incorporate the case casualty rate (CFR), which focuses on the extent of people with a specific case who passed on from that condition. The case-casualty proportion is an assessment of the seriousness of that condition. Although a massive loss of life has occurred, still, overall, the CFR of SARS-CoV-2 is lower than earlier variations, specifically SARS CoV-1 and MERS (Hawks et al., 2020; Shereen et al., 2020). The SARS-CoV-2 is zoonotic, and human-to-human transmission transformed this disease into a pandemic. The medical clinics' flood with patients having clinical manifestations of SARS-CoV-2 demonstrates the raised degree of human-to-human transmission rate (J. Xu et al., 2020). Since the day the principal contamination was affirmed, the number of tainted people proceeded consistently (Table 2) (Shereen et al., 2020). More than 220 countries have already reported confirmed cases all around the globe (Chan, Yuan, et al., 2020).

Table 2. Top 10 countries with the count of SARS-CoV-2 related cases, along with the total case count worldwide as of 27 July 2021.

Country	Total Cases	New Cases	Total Deaths	New Deaths	Total Recovered	Active Cases	Critical Cases
Worldwide	194,669,939	+296,849	4,172,559	+4552	176,662,440	13,834,940	84,074
USA	35,185,064	+393	626,717	+4	29,507,148	5,051,199	7771
India	31,396,300	+24,814	420,758	+173	30,555,315	420,227	8944
Brazil	19,670,534		549,500	-	18,340,760	780,274	8318
Russia	6,126,541	+24,072	153,874	+779	5,490,634	482,033	2300
France	5,697,912	-	111,616	-	5,674,587	192,492	878
UK	5,978,695	+29,173	129,158	+28	4,450,204	1,118,550	699
Turkey	5,587,378	-	50,879	-	5,415,937	120,562	543
Argentina	4,839,109	-	103,584	-	4,480,336	255,189	4318
Colombia	4,716,798	-	118,538	-	4,477,155	121,105	8155
Italy	4,317,415	+4,743	127,949	+7	4,123,209	66,257	178

Evidence revealed that intra-family and local area transmission is the potential triggering factor for the mass spread of the SARS-CoV-2 virus. Contamination might occur when people unconsciously come into contact with an infected individual who is sniffling, coughing, or releasing respiratory vapor through their nose or mouth (Alhumaid et al., 2021; Hossain, Ahmmed, Kuddus, et al., 2021; *Worldometer,2021*, n.d.-b). Even these droplets remain for a long period in the environment, and may cause infection to a person staying at a distance of more than a meter (Alhumaid et al., 2021). Still, more investigation is required to get a clear insight into the community transmission process of SARS-CoV-2 (Ong et al., 2020).

4.2 Fatality Rate of the Pandemic

Fatality rates can be an indicator of the disease severity and healthcare quality of an outbreak like COVID-19. By now, two distinguished criteria are used to facilitate the understanding of the death proportion of an infected population, namely infection fatality ratio (IFR) and case fatality ratio (CFR). The IFR is calculated by considering all the deaths against the total number of infected individuals. In comparison, CRF counts the death rate by dividing total deaths by individuals with confirmed cases. However, use of the term "rate" here is theoretically incorrect, as the "rate" assigns a time component, and the time factor lacks in CRF. Therefore, curators have proposed calling this the "case fatality proportion'' or "case fatality ratio''. The accurate estimation of the IFR and CFR depends upon the definite counting of infected people, and the number of deaths resulting from the disease. In the case of an ongoing pandemic like COVID-19, most of the fatality ratio records being conducted depend upon surveillance and crude tracking. Consequently, the CFR varies between countries, ranging from below 0.1% to over 25% (Ergönül et al., 2021; *WHO,2021*, n.d.-a) . The IFR and CFR equations recommended by WHO (*WHO,2021*, n.d.-a) are as follows:

$$\text{Infection fatality ratio (IFR, in \%)} = \frac{\text{Number of deaths from disease}}{\text{Number of infected individuals}} \times 100$$

$$\text{Case fatality ratio (IFR, in \%)} = \frac{\text{Number of deaths from disease}}{\text{Number of confirmed cases of disease}} \times 100$$

In the case of an ongoing pandemic, using the above-mentioned formula provides conditional CFR estimation due to reporting lag dates of the deaths and cases. As a result, the curated version (*WHO,2021*, n.d.-a) is as follows:

$$\text{Case fatality ratio (IFR, in \%)} = \frac{\text{Number of deaths from disease}}{\text{Number of deaths from disease+Number of recovered from disease}} \times 100$$

A study on laboratory-confirmed cases of COVID-19 declared the global CFR for Singapore to be from ~0.1% to ~6.9%, and from ~0.1% to ~16.3% in Belgium (*COVID-19 Map,2020*, n.d.) .Furthermore, CFR has been found to be low in people below 19 (0–0.1%) and from 20 to 54 (0.1–0.8%) years of age (W. Guan et al., 2020; 'Osong Public Health and Research Perspectives 2020', 2020).There is a significant rise in the CFR along with an increase in age, such as between 55 and 74 (1.4–4.9%) years, 75 and 84 (4.3–10.5%) years, and ≥85(10.4–27.3%) years (Bialek et al., 2020; R. Li et al., 2020). The situation was, surprisingly, more dreadful in patients with comorbidity, including diabetes, cardiovascular problems, threatening tumors, liver, and kidney-related intricacies, or bargained invulnerable systems (J. Gao et al., 2020). Additionally, weight and hypertension are reasons for higher CFR. Conversely, high COVID-19 testing facilities, healthcare facilities, and people living in rural areas are significantly less prone to CFR (Ergönül et al., 2021). Surprisingly, SARS-CoV-2 has comparatively lower CFR value than previous SARS CoV-1 (CFR 9.5%) and MERS (CFR 34.4%) (Rajgor et al., 2020). Furthermore, SARS-CoV-2 has a higher transmission ability with a Ro (reproduction rate) of about 2.5%, by WHO analysis (Hossain, 2020). Elevated values of Ro and CFR create more vulnerable and fragile situations for the healthcare system (Dong et al., 2020; Gharizadeh et al., 2021).

Chapter: 5

Pathogenesis Process of SARS CoV-2

5.1 Transmission

At first, the cases were identified with direct exposure to contaminated creatures (transmission from animal to human) at a fish market in Wuhan, China. After that, clinical cases with community transmission came to light. This supported the idea regarding a doable human-to-human transmission of the infection. In this way, human-to-human transmission is currently viewed as the principal type of transmission. The virus can also be transmitted from an asymptomatic person; yet, symptomatic individuals are the predominant transmission source. The transmission process begins with the passing of respiratory droplets via sneezing or coughing (Cascella et al., 2022). The study also reports that transmission can occur due to nearby interaction between individuals (Ghinai et al., 2020). Current statistics suggest three to seven days as the incubation period for the virus, whereas some studies depicted it to be closer to five days and the incubation time between 2 and 14 days (Ashour et al., 2020; Q et al., 2020; Rabaan, Al-Ahmed, Muhammad, et al., 2021; Uras, n.d.).These outcomes have been recorded from earlier cases. Therefore, advanced studies are required to track down transmission dynamics and incubation times (Hassan et al., 2020). Transmission can be traced down to the patient's natural liquids, for instance, respiratory beads, spit, excrement, and pee (Bari et al., 2021). The most appropriate temperature for virion endurance demonstrates that 22 °C has a less noteworthy endurance rate than 4 °C (Kampf et al., 2020; Otter et al., 2016). As SARS-CoV-2 virions are held all throughout the clinical course, patients with asymptomatic symptoms of COVID-19 can spread the disease as well, during the indicative course, and at the hour of the clinical recuperation time frame. Furthermore, additional alerts ought to be kept up during the endurance time of the SARS-CoV-2 virions on a superficial level. SARS-CoV-2 infection half-life on copper, vaporizers, cardboard, hardened steel, and plastic surfaces are 1, 1.5, 3.4, 5.6, and 6.8 h individually, as per the information given by specific tests (van Doremalen et al., 2020, p. 1).

5.2 Pathological Process

Although β coronavirus shows a higher species conservancy than the other coronavirus families, the minor mutation in its genome can suddenly change to its pathogenicity, tissue tropism, and host range. The introduction of this zoonotic disease (SARS CoVs and MERS) into the human chronicle provides an indisputable sign of adaptability of these virus particles (Peiris et al., 2004; Zaki et al., 2012). There is a censorious role played by the median hosts that completes the cross-species transmission process, and this is important at the same time for building the connection between the virus and the new hosts to facilitate the viral replication process in a new environment (Brennan et al., 2014).

In order to limit the quick pervasiveness of SARS-CoV-2, immediate surveillance is required to monitor its further host adaptation, transmissibility, infectivity, viral evolution, and pathogenicity. The receptor and multiple molecular interactions are some of the modulating factors for the viral host range. Regardless of the difference between the SARS CoV and SARS-CoV-2, structural similarity was found in their spike protein's receptor-binding domain (RBD) (R. Lu et al., 2020). Moreover, critical residues such as Asn501 and Gln493 modulate the interaction between the ACE2 from host receptors and RBD of SARS-CoV-2, which ultimately facilitates the person-to-person transmission process (Wan et al., n.d.).

5.3 Host Response

SARS-CoV-2 adopts a dodgy mechanism to escape the host's innate immune response and successfully infect healthy individuals. Since SARS-CoV-2 and SARS-CoV show close clinical manifestations, SARS-CoV-2 has unique pathogenesis and biochemical processes comparable to SARS CoV (Huang et al., 2020). Following SARS-CoV infections, the release of IFN-stimulated genes (ISGs) induced by the type I interferon (IFN) occurs against the viral replication process. In response to this defense activity by host cells, SARS-CoV-2 secretes a minimum of eight antagonizing factors that neutralize the ISG's activity (Totura & Baric, 2012). However, the immune response mediated by the host's defense system poses a critical role in limiting viral dissemination. Nevertheless, excess promptness of the immune cells, coupled with lytic stress by viral invasion, results in severe disease outcomes. The most common symptoms manifested at the early stage include patients with acute body pain, pneumonia, dry cough, and fever (Huang et al., 2020; Rakib et al., 2021). Further progress rapidly results in acute respiratory stress syndrome (ARDS), septic shock, and organ failure, followed by death (Rakib et al., 2021). After COVID-19 infection, the development of ARDS and the subsequent damages occurring at the alveolar type II pulmonary cells as well as in the ciliated epithelium cells of the airways suggest that ACE2 is abundant in lung cells, acting as a gateway for virus entry (Hamming et al., 2004). A similar mode of the inflammatory cascade has been reported in both SARS-CoV-2 and SARS-CoV infected patients. A bulk load of pro-inflammatory cytokines (e.g., interleukin (IFN-γ, IFN-γ-induced protein 10 (IP10), IL-1, IL-6, IL-12)), monocyte chemoattractant protein-1 (MCP1), and macrophage inflammatory proteins1A (MIP1A) were found in serum collected from previously infected patients with SARS-CoV. These immune cells are also related to severe lung damage and pulmonary inflammation (WONG et al., 2004). In addition, a high level of pro-inflammatory cytokines such as TNF-α, IL1β, IL-2, IL7, and MCP1were found in samples of SARS-CoV-2 infected patients. On the other hand, (ICU) intensive care unit patients of COVID-19 contained a greater load of cytokines such as TNF-α, GSCF, MCP1, and IP10 compared to the non-ICU patients. This suggests that cytokine storms can be the underlying cause of severe disease manifestation (R. Lu et al., 2020). The study reports that a high cytokine concentration has a reversible correlation with the total immune cell (T, CD4+, and CD8+) counts in SARS-CoV-2 infection. Hence, lower T cell counts can be a potential biomarker for risk stratification of patients infected with COVID-19 (Diao et al., 2020). Besides, other findings reported that adults (males) are more vulnerable to SARS-CoV-2 infection than young children (Huang et al., 2020; Rakib et al., 2021). A similar finding was observed in the experiment on a primate model called Cynomolgus macaque (crab-eating monkey) (Smits et al., 2010). Further follow-up studies are warranted from the scientific community to get a better understanding of the virulence factors of SARS-CoV-2 (Kakodkar et al., 2020).

Chapter: 6

Post-Infection Outcomes

6.1 Clinical Features

Clinical signs of SARS-CoV-2 infection have close likenesses with SARS-CoV, where the most well-known indications incorporate fever, dry hack, dyspnea, chest torment, exhaustion, and myalgia (J. Chen, 2020; R. Lu et al., 2020). Less continuous signs include migraine, unsteadiness, stomach torment, loose bowels, queasiness, and regurgitating (R. Lu et al., 2020; Yan et al., 2020). Given the data of the first 425 affirmed cases from Wuhan, the most well-known signs incorporate fever, dry hack, myalgia, and weariness. Then again, more uncommon side effects are sputum creation, migraine, hemoptysis, stomach torment, and looseness of the bowels **(Table 3)** (Paules et al., 2020). Around 75% of patients have bilateral pneumonia (de Wit et al., 2016). Apart from SARS-CoV and MERS viral infections, COVID-19 patients display noteworthy upper respiratory tract symptoms, including sore throat, rhinorrhea, and sneezing (R. Lu et al., 2020). Extreme inconveniences and intricacies, such as hypoxemia, intense ARDS, arrhythmia, stun, severe cardiovascular damage, and serious renal damage, have been noted in COVID-19 patients (de Wit et al., 2016; R. Lu et al., 2020). A study of 99 patients revealed that approximately 17% of patients displayed ARDS, and 11% of patients died of several organ failures (de Wit et al., 2016). The median time from onset of symptoms to ARDS is eight days (Rakib et al., 2020, p.).

Table 3. Clinical manifestations and laboratory-based findings of a patient with SARS-CoV-2 viral infection.

	Outcomes	Percentage (%)
Common signs and symptoms	Fever	77.4–98.6%
	Cough	59.4–81.8%
	Fatigue	38.1–69.6%
	Dyspnea	3.2–55.0%
	Myalgia	11.1–34.8%
	Sputum production	28.2–56.5%
	Headache	6.5–33.9%
	Underlying diseases	25.2–50.5%
	Lymphopenia	35.3–82.1%

Laboratory outcomes	Thrombocytopenia	5.0–36.2%
	Leukopenia	9.1–33.7%
	Increased CRP	60.7–86.3%
	Increased D-dimer	36.4–46.4%
	Increased LDH	27.4–75.8%
	Increased CK	8.0–32.5%
	Prolonged prothrombin time	58.0%
	Increased ALT	16.1–28.3%
	Increased AST	22.2–36.7%
	Increased interleukin-6	51.5%
	Increased serum ferritin	62.6%
	Increased ESR	84.8%
	Increased procalcitonin	5.5–11.3%
	Increased troponin I	12.2%
	Increased creatinine	1.9–9.8%
Complications and fatality	ARDS	3.4–29.3%
	Shock	1.0–8.7%
	Acute renal injury	0.5–7.3%
	Acute cardiac injury	7.2–12.2%
	Secondary infections	9.8%

6.2 Disease Prognosis

Reports from the study based on a large number of positive cases of COVID-19, especially the severely ill patients, found complications such as ARDS, acute cardiac injury, acute renal injury, shock, and secondary infection. The fatality rate due to COVID-19 infection fluctuated from 0 to 14.6% (Bai et al., 2020, p. 1; Huang et al., 2020; Rabaan, Al-Ahmed, Garout, et al., 2021; Rakib et al., 2021, p. 2; X.-W. Xu et al., 2020). A comparative data analysis between the ICU patients and the non-ICU patients showed that most aged adults with comorbidities occupied the ICU and had more frequent abdominal pain, anorexia, and dyspnea (Bai et al., 2020, p. 1). Concurrently, it is suggested that patients in ICU deposited a bulk amount of chemokine and plasma cytokines that include TNFα, GSCF, MCP1, MIP1A, IL2, IL7, IL10, and IP10 (Huang et al., 2020). Conversely, the non-surviving patients develop more acute lymphopenia and enriched levels of neutrophil, d-dimer, and fibrin derogation products than the surviving individuals (Bai et al., 2020, p. 1; Z. Xu et al., 2020). As of 22 January 2020, an analysis conducted on 17 death cases of COVID-19 by Wang et al. found that the median days from the onset of early symptoms until death were 14.0 (range 6–41) days, and consistently appeared to be shorter for older individuals (Wang et al., 2020). Symptoms such as abdominal pain and dyspnea, comorbidities, age, and significant clinical anomalies (elevated d-dimer, lymphopenia, etc.) may all lead to the risk of poor outcomes (**Table 4)** (Bai et al., 2020, p. 19; Wang et al., 2020; Yang et al., 2020; J. Zhang, Dong, et al., 2020). However, SARS-CoV-2 has a comparatively lower mortality rate than SARS-CoV and MERS (Ge et al., 2020, p. 19; Zumla et al., 2015).

Table 4. Risk factors associated with COVID-19 patients.

Risk Factors	**Aftermath**
Age	Adults (65–84) years make up estimated COVID-19 deaths of (4–11%) in the U.S, while adults ages 85 and above make up 10–27%.
Diabetes (type 1 and type 2)	People with diabetes were nearly 3.7 times more likely to have a critical case of COVID-19 or die from the disease.
Heart disease and hypertension	People with conditions that affect the cardiovascular system, such as heart disease and hypertension, generally suffer worse complications of COVID-19.
Smoking	Smokers face a heightened risk of developing pneumonia, suffering organ damage, and requiring breathing support.
Blood group type	People with blood types of A group (A-positive, A-negative, and AB-positive, AB-negative) were at a higher risk of contracting the disease compared with non-A-group types.
Obesity	Obese COVID-19 patients were more than twice as likely to develop severe pneumonia as compared to patients who were of normal weight.
Genetic factors	Genes for ACE2 receptors in patient's body make it easier getting infected by COVID-19.

Chapter: 7

Diagnostic Strategies for COVID-19

To track down the disease severity, complicated detection methods are inevitable. There are two types of diagnosis methods—(1) molecular or viral test and (2) serological or antibody test (*Johns Hopkins Coronavirus Resource Center*, n.d.). The molecular tests involve the testing of a nasopharyngeal (NP) swab or oropharyngeal (OP) swab, stool, sputum, or bronchoalveolar lavage for the existence of viral RNA. However, the FDA suggests patients' sputum for testing in the laboratory as an "Emergency Use Authorization" (*Johns Hopkins Coronavirus Resource Center*, n.d.). WHO prescribed that samples be collected from both lower and upper respiratory tracts (Hassan et al., 2020). The molecular test consists of two types, the (1) PCR test and (2) antigen test. Additionally, a serology test involves tracing antibodies in blood samples to ensure prior viral infection of a patient (West et al., 2021). Molecular tests provide the utmost accuracy relative to other detection methods (Hoque et al., 2020). Combining both of the methods gradually increases the detection sensitivity ($p < 0.001$) (Shormin & Yusuf, 2020). The FDA has authorized two hundred manufacturers for molecular tests and 50 manufacturers for serological tests (*GoodRx Health*, n.d.). Serology tests can be executed as an elective identification approach on the off chance that the sub-atomic test is inaccurate; however, both of the discovery techniques have a few downsides. The sub-atomic perceptibility may be diminished due to inappropriate sample handling or issues incurred when blood tests are performed before the principal seven-day stretch of the disease. Serology test results will be flawed when not performed at the appropriate time, since IgM does not appear until seven days after infection and IgG until 15 days (Shormin & Yusuf, 2020). RT-PCR is a foremost testing technique that utilizes warm cycling to create about 35 billion DNA duplicates from RNA records. Fluorescent color is utilized to recognize the presence of target tests. The outcome is positive after it arrives at a specific cycle limit (Ct-esteem). For the same RT-PCR, another atomic procedure RT-LAMP (Reverse Transcriptional Loop-Mediated Isothermal Amplification) uses a similar method. However, rather than applying a progression of various temperature cycles, like RT-PCR, it prompts a steady temperature size of around (60–65) °C. The uniqueness of this technique is that it very well may be estimated with unaided eyes, since a compound called "magnesium pyrophosphate" makes an overcast shading. Simultaneously, serological tests including ELISA and lateral flow measures distinguish antigens and neutralizers in blood tests (Kile et al.,2021.). Besides, computerized tomography (CT) can be a compensative choice for the deficit of RT-PCR technology. An experimental report from Wuhan depicts that CT images referred to 98% detection sensitivity compared to RT-PCR (78%). CT images have also been used in Turkey because of test kit shortage (Fang et al., 2020). However, cell culture is not recommended due to its numerous drawbacks. Additionally, CRISPR-Cas mediated technology can become another potential diagnostic method over time (Hoque et al., 2020).

Chapter: 8

Prevention against COVID-19

8.1 Preventive Measures

The shock of Severe Acute Respiratory Syndrome Coronavirus (SARS-CoV) in 2002 and the Middle East Respiratory Syndrome Coronavirus (MERS-CoV) in 2012 were viewed as the most effective variation of COVIDs until the emergence of COVID-19, the third novel Covid to cause a wide-scale scourge in the 21st century (Alanagreh et al., 2020). COVID-19 has far stronger transmissibility compared to prior variants, causing emergent outbreaks throughout the world. Though COVID-19 has been considered a category "B" infectious disease by law, it is being treated and handled as a category "A" contagious disease due to its rapid transmissibility. Transmission root impeding, source controlling, and protecting susceptive people can effectively impede the illness' severity (Shen et al., 2020). The spread of COVID-19 can be limited by agreeing with the accompanying rules given by WHO to the worldwide populace, which include the following: (*WHO,2021*, n.d.)

- Optimizing infection control protocols, self-isolation, and isolated accommodation for patients.
- Immunocompromised, aged persons must take special care; health care personnel must use PPE such as N95, FFP3 mask, gowns, face shield, etc.
- Frequent handwashing with soap and water, with hand sanitizer as an alternative disinfection process; alcohol can also be used.
- Avoid public gatherings and maintain social distancing of at least 1 m. Must wear face masks and cover coughs and sneezes to help prevent aerosol transmission.

Public health measures are daily precautionary activities that include:

- All of us should put on face masks and maintain respiratory and hand hygiene.
- Staying home during sickness.
- Covering mouth and nose with bent elbow or tissue at the time of sneezing or coughing. Used tissue should be disposed of instantly.
- Washing hands regularly with soap and water. Hand hygiene refers to the use of alcohol-based hand sanitizers before and after each patient's contact as well as after touching any surface, transport, money, etc. Washing hands with soapy water for 20 s is also very

effective and essential for everyone. It is also advised to maintain hand hygiene before and after cooking, before eating, before and after removing gloves and face masks, and after using the toilet. Distinct reusable utensils can be used by the patient after proper cleaning.

- Avoiding handshaking is also advised for the time being for your protection.
- Cleaning regularly touched surfaces and objects. Disinfecting the surrounding environment of the patient, including toilet and furniture. Clean and disinfect bathroom and toilet surfaces at least once every day. Regular household soap or detergent should be used first for cleaning and rinsing purposes; regular household disinfectant and germ killer containing 0.5% sodium hypochlorite (NaOCl) should be applied (World Health Organization, 2020).
- Provisionally, prevention is the best way to stop the spread of infection. WHO has boldly recommended hand and respiratory hygiene for cases, contacts, and health care workers (WHO, 2020b).
- The medical musk is not needed for the general public, excluding doctors and people associated with the health care system. Patients and caregivers are recommended to remove the mask from behind and practice hand hygiene after removing it (World Health Organization, 2020).
- The doctors and health workers are particularly advised to wear personal protective equipment (PPE), including an N95 respirator mask and eye shield, while collecting respiratory samples. Avoiding contact with body fluids is mandatory (WHO, 2020a).
- The duration of quarantine is 14 days from the last contact with PCR confirmed COVID-19 case. They should be checked daily for fever and other symptoms associated with COVID-19.
- Children's health monitoring is necessary during this time. Children with a history of close contact with infected patients need to be routinely observed for body temperature and clinical features. When presenting with doubtful symptoms, children should be taken to a delegated hospital for screening. Newborns delivered by COVID-19 infected mothers must complete a pathogen test and be isolated in a single cabin room or at home according to their medical conditions (Shen et al., 2020).

8.2 Treatment

As new immunizations are intermittently gaining endorsement, this doesn't guarantee accessibility, nor the adequacy of the antibodies. Experts assume that around 90% of individuals of lower-income nations will be denied immunization until 2023 or later. At the same time, immunization aversion in wealthier countries like the USA may transform this into an even more mind-boggling circumstance. Subsequently, even though immunizations are continuously being provided locally, this is no time to overlook security measures (individual cleanliness, face masks, social separating) (Su et al., 2021). However, researchers are trying to globally defend against this virus attack with every possible means. After a comprehensive literature review, we categorized the whole treatment approach into two major groups: (1) physiological treatment and (2) mediated treatment **(Figure 6)**. The physiological treatment mainly involves monitoring viral symptoms and providing equipment support (oxygen saturation, balanced water-electrolyte level, balanced diet, etc.) (Hanna et al., 2021).

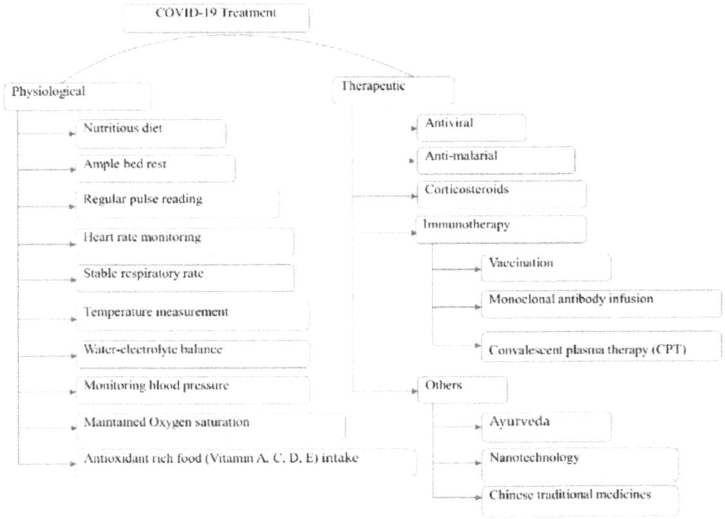

Figure 6. Overview of the possible COVID-19 treatment measures.

Coronavirus patient management depends upon steady estimates that incorporate ventilation, liquid administration, oxygenation, low–portion antiviral complex, and interferon inward breath (Cunningham et al., 2020; Rc, 2020). The significant commitment before intensive treatment is to confine any presumed patients in a different room, as per the specialist's proposal. Basic cases are promptly take to the ICU. The resulting treatment course includes sufficient bed rest, consuming sufficient water and calories, and guaranteeing sufficient oxygen immersion (Dg et al., 2020, p. 19; Shen et al., 2020). A study suggests that mildly symptomatic patients can be treated at home by providing standard care, including an adequate supply of proper nutrition, hydration, fever, and cold management. For patients with fatigue and a temperature above 38.5 °C, it is recommended to provide a lukewarm water bath and antipyretic drug therapy. However, routine medication with antibiotics and anti-viral drugs is highly prohibited (Dg et al., 2020). Along with supportive treatment, some potential COVID treatments have been tested in trials, listed in **Table 5**.

Table 5. Different approaches of prospective therapeutic trials against nCoV-19.

Host	Ref.
Human human Vero E6 cells Human Human Human	(Cunningham et al., 2020; Hossain, Jannat, Brishty, et al., 2021; McCreary et al., 2020)
Vero E6 cells Human	(McCreary et al., 2020; Rosa & Santos, 2020)
Human	(Hanna et al., 2021)
Human	(Guaraldi et al., 2020; Hossain & Rahman, 2021; Lan et al., 2020; Toniati et al., 2020)

Treatment	Drugs	Function	Dose
Anti-viral	Oseltamivir	No activity	75 mg every 12 h (orally)
	Ganciclovir	-	0.25 g every 12 h (IV)
	Remdesivir	Inhibits coronavirus replication including SARS-CoV-2.	0.77 μM 48 h
	Lopinavir/Ritonavir	Blocks the main protease of SARS-CoV-1 and inhibits viral replication	400/100 mg twice daily
	Arbidol (Umifenovir)	No clinical data are available	200 mg Orally 3 times
	Interferon-α (IFN-α)	Reduces infection rate	500 mg ribavirin combined (2–3) times a day
Anti- malarial	Chloroquine	1. Anti-viral and anti-inflammatory activities and 2. Post translation alteration by glycosylation inhibition.	1.13 μM 48 h
	Hydroxyl chloroquine		200 mg every 8 h (orally)
Cortico steroids	Methyl prednisolone	-	1–2 mg/kg·d For 3 days (IV)
Immune therapy	Convalescent Plasma therapy (CPT)	-	200–500 mL
	Tocilizumab (Atlizumap) mAb	Anti-interleukin-6 receptor activity	400 mg (For body weight < 75 kg) Or 600 mg (For body weight ≥ 75 kg)max dose 800 mg Repeat after 12 h if required (IV)
	Anakinra	Anti-interleukin-1β neutralizing	100 mg twice a day for 72 h and later on single dose per day for 7 days

Moreover, repurposing of existing antiviral medications, including lopinavir, ritonavir, chloroquine, interferon beta, and remdesivir, has been launched as an international clinical trial by the WHO SOLIDARITY trial project (Uddin et al., 2020). However, these medication trials could not provide any reliable remedy, and two of the reports rejected the use of these antiviral drugs

(Mahmud et al., 2021). Surprisingly, remdesivir has been proved to be efficient for severe patients with increased ventilation and proved to be less risky (Young et al., 2021).

Moreover, another multidimensional approach for COVID-19 treatment involves 5000-year-old traditional Chinese medicine (TCM), including Huoxiang Zhengqi, Lianhua Qingwen, Shufeng Jiedu, and Xue Bijing used as pills, powder, tea, or tincture, which was proven to be effective in 2002 against the SARS-CoV infection at an early stage by increasing patients' oxyhemoglobin arterial saturation (Rosa & Santos, 2020; Tong et al., 2020, p. 19). Furthermore, the intake of antioxidant-rich foods containing Vitamin A, C, D, and E can mitigate the damage via oxidation as well as the risk of cardiovascular disease (Hanna et al., 2021). Additionally, curcumin, honey, omega-3 fatty acids, and potato starch have some natural anti-inflammatory activities (Hanna et al., 2021; Zahedipour et al., 2020). On March 16 of 2020, Regeneron Pharmaceuticals Inc., US, and Sanofi collaboratively announced the phase 2 and 3 clinical trials of a human monoclonal antibody called Sarilumab (Kevzara) against the interleukin-6 (IL-6) receptor on about 400 hospitalized corona patients (Hossain, Jannat, Brishty, et al., 2021, p. 19). On the other hand, a study showed the prophylaxis potential of Tocilizumab (humanized monoclonal antibody) and Melatonin (N-acetyl-5-methoxytryptamine) as two candidate molecules for nCoV-19 treatment (McCreary et al., 2020; R. Zhang, Wang, et al., 2020). Other potential COVID-19 treatments may include nanotechnology, nitric oxide (NO), CRISPR/Cas13d System, Yoga, and Ayurveda (Mir & Maurya, 2021; Z. Tang et al., 2021; Tillu et al., 2020)(Hanna et al., 2021)

8.3 Vaccination

As of now, vaccination is considered a definitive encapsulation comparative with any remaining existing solutions for COVID-19 outbreak. Researchers universally are working next to each other, utilizing accessible innovation and labor to beat this pandemic (Hanna et al., 2021; Hossain, Kuddus, Rashid, et al., 2021). This overall process may need around 12 to 18 months for achieving promising outcomes and high throughput manufacturing (Stockman et al., 2006). By now, mainly the mRNA, epitopes, and spike protein RBD (receptor binding domain) structure-based vaccine initiatives are being proposed **(Table 6)** (Scagnolari et al., 2004). At present, 98 vaccines are being evaluated on humans clinically, 32 are in their last phase of the trial, and a minimum of 77 vaccines are in their active preclinical animal trial (*New York Times*, n.d.). Several leading vaccine candidates were listed in **Table 6** according to the data of 27 July 2021.

Table 6. Top 10 leading vaccine candidates with their efficacy level worldwide as of 27 July 2021(*New York Times*, n.d.) .

Dose	Phase	Efficacy	Approved in countries
2 doses (Three-weeks apart)	2/3	91.3%	Bahrain, Brazil, New Zealand, Saudi Arabia, Switzerland
2 doses (Four-weeks apart)	3	Over 90%	Switzerland
2 doses (Three-weeks apart)	3	91.6%	Russia (Emergency use)
2 doses	2/3	76%	Brazil
Single dose	3	65.28%	China
Single dose	3	72% (U.S.A.); 68% (Brazil); 64% (South Africa)	USA (Emergency use)
2 doses (Three-weeks apart)	3	Unknown	Turkmenistan
2 doses (Three-weeks apart)	3	89.7%	N/A
2 doses (Three-weeks apart)	3	78%	Bahrain, UAE, China
2 doses (Two-weeks apart)	3	50.65% (Brazil trial) 83.5% (Turkey trial)	China

Vaccine Name	Developer	Technology
Comirnaty or Tozinameran or BNT162b2	Pfizer and BioNTech	mRNA
mRNA1273 or Spikevax	Moderna	mRNA
Sputnik V or Gam-Covid-Vac)	Gamaleya Research Institute	Ad5, Ad26 (Adenovirus)
Vaxzevria or AZD1222 (also known as Covishield in India)	University of Oxford and the British-Swedish company AstraZeneca	ChAdOx1
Convidecia (also known as Ad5-nCoV)	CanSino Biologics and Institute of Biology, Academy of Military Medical Sciences	Ad5(Adenovirus)
Ad26.COV2.S	Johnson & Johnson Beth Israel Deaconess Medical Center	Ad26(Adenovirus)
EpiVacCorona	Vector Institute	Protein
NVX-CoV2373	Novavax	Protein
BBIBP-CorV	Sinopharm	Inactivated
CoronaVac (formerly PiCoVacc)	Sinovac Biotech	Inactivated

The vaccine pillar of the ACT, COVAX, is co-led by Gavi (the Coalition for Epidemic Preparedness Innovations) and WHO. It is formed to maintain the pace of vaccine development and production and ensure the equal distribution of the vaccine, so that no low-income country lags in vaccination. COVAX set a target of vaccine supply that can compensate a minimum of 20% of the country's population (*COVAX*, n.d.). At this point, AstraZeneca has agreed to provide vaccines to COVAX, whereas Moderna and Pfizer have not yet confirmed anything. On the other hand, there are also some vital issues relating to the mass supply and conservation of the vaccines in remote places, including cold-chain requirements, logistics, and delays, which has made the situation more challenging (Kim et al., 2021).

8.4 Boosting Immunity

Boosting resistance includes measures like a reasonable eating regimen, standard exercise, maintaining a strategic distance from additional pressure and weariness, oral wellbeing, and sufficient rest, that are significant not just in forestalling different contaminations, like viral assault, but also in maintaining mental and psychological wellness. Organic citrus products containing Vitamin C (ascorbic corrosive) and different nutrients can stimulate the insusceptible framework, as well. Overall, inoculation is the most essential step to protect against the resistant triggers of a viral assault like SARS-CoV-2 (Shen et al., 2020).

Chapter: 9

Infection Associated Factors

9.1 Gender Biases

The reports from different case study data indicate a clear contrast between men and women, especially in the case of mortality and other disease outcomes (Wenham et al., 2020, p. 1). Studies governed in China and Italy showed that the mortality rate in men is much higher than in women (Kocher et al., 2021; Rakib et al., 2021; X.-C. Tang et al., 2014). The higher ACE2 receptor expression in the lungs of men compared to women can be a causative factor for this (S. P et al., 2020). Moreover, the risk appears higher in men in their 50s and starts to mitigate in the 90s. In China, the mortality rate for men and women was 2.8% and 1.7%, respectively (Kocher et al., 2021). The exact reasons behind the gendered impact of COVID-19 remain unsolved, although behavioral and genetic factors could be plausible indicators for this (Wenham et al., 2020). Reasons why men may possess greater susceptibility to COVID-19 relative to the female population may include a higher smoking rate in men, sex-based immunological variance, and a higher portion of comorbidity (hypertension, heart disease) in men (Kocher et al., 2021).

9.2 Ethnic Differences

The COVID-19 effects on various ethnic groups are affected fundamentally by the aberrations between medical care availability and financial status. Lower financial conditions and a raised pace of comorbidity impact the COVID-19 withdrawal (Kopel et al., 2020, p.). In March 2020, The CDC and COVID-19–Associated Hospitalization Surveillance Network conducted a study on 580 hospitalized COVID-19 patients with ethnicity data from 14 states in the US. This study found that, among the patients, about 45.0% were Caucasian (~76% of the US population), 33% were African-American (~13% of the US population), 8% Hispanic (~18% of the US population), and the remainder consisted of 5% Asian, less than 1% American Indian/Alaskan Native, and 7.9% from unknown or other races. However, the racial distribution varied by state depending on the target population size. It has been noted that smaller populations like African Americans have greater COVID-19 infection risk as they are much more prone to have heart disease, asthma, obesity, hypertension, and diabetes (Garg et al., 2020). Moreover, minority populations also possess a higher number of people with low socio-economic conditions, contributing to the risk of COVID-19 contraction. A prior investigation on CytoMegalo Virus (CMV) found a significant relationship between cell-mediated immunity and low socio-economic status among different socio-economic populations in the USA, suggesting that people with poor socio-economic condition have access to fewer healthcare facilities, greater life stressors, and a poorer diet, which results in a weak immune system (Adler et al., 1993; Dowd & Aiello, 2009; Steptoe et al., 2007). On the other hand, higher ACE2 receptor expression in Asian people than in the African American and Caucasian populations may cause dispersed outcomes across different countries (S. P et al., 2020).

9.3 Environmental Effect

Viruses do not replicate outside of a living cell, yet the infectious viruses may continue on infected natural surfaces, and the span of an active infection is obviously controlled by certain ecological boundaries, for example, temperature and moistness (Chowdhury et al., 2021). Dirty surfaces are significant vectors in the infection transmission measure in medical clinic conditions, just as in the local area. A recent study reported that surfaces and suspensions could be recognized as potential transmission sources that might lead to hospital-acquired infections with human coronavirus (Chowdhury et al., 2021). The environmental sustainability of SARS-CoV-2 was previously unknown. However, various studies have demonstrated that SARS CoV can withstand at least two weeks in dry conditions. The dried-out virus on smooth surfaces maintains its viability for more than five days at a temperature of 22–25 °C and relative humidity of 40–50%. The virus remains constant for three weeks at room temperature in a fluid environment, but it is easily killed by heat treatment at 56 °C for 15 min (*Severe Acute Respiratory Syndrome (SARS)*, n.d.). However, virus viability was quickly lost when temperature and humidity were relatively higher (38 °C, and relative humidity of >95%). This indicates that SARS-CoV-2 is a stable virus that may be transmitted through indirect contact or fomites (Seto et al., 2003). Such consequences may allude to the significant role of contaminated surfaces in pathogen transmission in the hospital and the community. SARS-CoV-2 is relatively firmer and steadier than the human coronaviruses 229E or OC43, and some other viral respiratory pathogens, such as a respiratory syncytial virus. Generally, direct droplet transmission is an important route of transmission (Seto et al., 2003). The robust stability of SARS coronavirus at low temperature and in a low humidity environment may allow for its rapid community transmission in subtropical areas (such as Hong Kong) during the spring season. These findings may also explain the reason why some Asian nations in equatorial areas (for example, Malaysia, Indonesia, or Thailand) with high temperatures and relatively humid environments did not have strong community outbreaks of the SARS virus compared to European regions (Sefren Geiner et al., 2020).

9.4 Blood Group and Coronavirus

A study indicates that people having blood group A is related to greater danger of disease by COVID-19 contrasted with non-A blood groups, while blood group O was connected with a similarly lower risk of contamination than non-O blood groups (Ellinghaus et al., 2020). Ensuing investigation showed that A positive individuals are at a 45%increased respiratory danger, though individuals with blood group O are at a 35% diminished likelihood of having respiratory complications. Late, an Italian–Spanish genome-wide affiliation examination-based investigation uncovered the linkage between blood groups and coronavirus (Ellinghaus et al., 2020). The effect of age and gender on the ABO blood group distribution in patients with novel coronavirus from two distinct hospitals was analyzed. The results concluded that age and gender do not impact the blood group (Zhao et al., 2021). However, interestingly, the consequence is significant for A and O blood group type only when the Rh factor is positive in blood samples (Zietz et al., 2020).

Chapter: 10

Future thoughts on COVID-19

The current COVID-19 pandemic situation has indeed affected the whole world, socially and economically. The world is now on the move to compensate for the damage done by COVID-19, and to fight back by developing vaccines, many of which are already being delivered globally. However, it should be noted that vaccines are effective only when vaccination is governed properly. Equity distribution to the lower-income countries and willing participation towards vaccination should be maintained to eradicate this crisis. Despite the vaccines' release, the global population should regularly practice personal hygiene, face masking, and social distancing until the vaccines are proved fully functional and available globally. However, the minimization of the huge load on the healthcare system and the growing mortality rate are two major problems currently receiving global efforts. The lesson taught by COVID-19 should be remembered for a long time, and advanced preparation is needed for any further global hazards that can put global health at stake. Furthermore, paying considerable attention to the plausible cause of this virus' transmission, there should be a total restriction on trading wild creatures and birds as a food source across the globe, and further investigations on SARS-CoV-2 genomic makeup must be carried out to understand its pathogenicity, epidemiology, and transmission pattern. Disclosing the genomic construction can provide insight into effective drug design and vaccine construction for subsequent variants. Artificial intelligence (AI) could also be an excellent tool to track down the transmission pattern of a deadly virus before it turns into an outbreak. Therefore, uninterrupted surveillance and proper coordination between national and international health stakeholders can balance the situation. Since the advancement in technology gave us the liberty to utilize our utmost potential to contribute to the betterment of human civilization, so this should be the time to make the best use of it.

References

Adler, N. E., Boyce, W. T., Chesney, M. A., Folkman, S., & Syme, S. L. (1993). Socioeconomic inequalities in health. No easy solution. *JAMA*, *269*(24), 3140–3145.

Alanagreh, L., Alzoughool, F., & Atoum, M. (2020). The Human Coronavirus Disease COVID-19: Its Origin, Characteristics, and Insights into Potential Drugs and Its Mechanisms. *Pathogens*, *9*(5), 331. https://doi.org/10.3390/pathogens9050331

Al-Horani, R. A., & Kar, S. (2020). Potential Anti-SARS-CoV-2 Therapeutics That Target the Post-Entry Stages of the Viral Life Cycle: A Comprehensive Review. *Viruses*, *12*(10), E1092. https://doi.org/10.3390/v12101092

Al-Horani, R. A., Kar, S., & Aliter, K. F. (2020). Potential Anti-COVID-19 Therapeutics that Block the Early Stage of the Viral Life Cycle: Structures, Mechanisms, and Clinical Trials. *International Journal of Molecular Sciences*, *21*(15), E5224. https://doi.org/10.3390/ijms21155224

Alhumaid, S., Al Mutair, A., Al Alawi, Z., Alsuliman, M., Ahmed, G. Y., Rabaan, A. A., Al-Tawfiq, J. A., & Al-Omari, A. (2021). Knowledge of infection prevention and control among healthcare workers and factors influencing compliance: A systematic review. *Antimicrobial Resistance and Infection Control*, *10*(1), 86. https://doi.org/10.1186/s13756-021-00957-0

Ashour, H. M., Elkhatib, W. F., Rahman, M. M., & Elshabrawy, H. A. (2020). Insights into the Recent 2019 Novel Coronavirus (SARS-CoV-2) in Light of Past Human Coronavirus Outbreaks. *Pathogens (Basel, Switzerland)*, *9*(3), E186. https://doi.org/10.3390/pathogens9030186

Atri, D., Siddiqi, H. K., Lang, J. P., Nauffal, V., Morrow, D. A., & Bohula, E. A. (2020). COVID-19 for the Cardiologist: Basic Virology, Epidemiology, Cardiac Manifestations, and Potential Therapeutic Strategies. *JACC: Basic to Translational Science*, *5*(5), 518–536. https://doi.org/10.1016/j.jacbts.2020.04.002

Bai, Y., Yao, L., Wei, T., Tian, F., Jin, D.-Y., Chen, L., & Wang, M. (2020). Presumed Asymptomatic Carrier Transmission of COVID-19. *JAMA*, *323*(14), 1406–1407. https://doi.org/10.1001/jama.2020.2565

Bari, M. S., Hossain, M. J., Akhter, S., & Emran, T. B. (2021). Delta variant and black fungal invasion: A bidirectional assault might worsen the massive second/third stream of COVID-19 outbreak in South-Asia. *Ethics, Medicine and Public Health*, *19*, 100722. https://doi.org/10.1016/j.jemep.2021.100722

Bar-On, Y. M., Flamholz, A., Phillips, R., & Milo, R. (2020). SARS-CoV-2 (COVID-19) by the numbers. *ELife*, *9*, e57309. https://doi.org/10.7554/eLife.57309

Belouzard, S., Chu, V. C., & Whittaker, G. R. (2009). Activation of the SARS coronavirus spike protein via sequential proteolytic cleavage at two distinct sites. *Proceedings of the National Academy of Sciences of the United States of America*, *106*(14), 5871–5876. https://doi.org/10.1073/pnas.0809524106

Benvenuto, D., Angeletti, S., Giovanetti, M., Bianchi, M., Pascarella, S., Cauda, R., Ciccozzi, M., & Cassone, A. (2020). Evolutionary analysis of SARS-CoV-2: How mutation of Non-Structural Protein 6 (NSP6) could affect viral autophagy. *The Journal of Infection*, *81*(1), e24–e27. https://doi.org/10.1016/j.jinf.2020.03.058

Benvenuto, D., Giovanetti, M., Salemi, M., Prosperi, M., De Flora, C., Junior Alcantara, L. C., Angeletti, S., & Ciccozzi, M. (2020). The global spread of 2019-nCoV: A molecular evolutionary analysis. *Pathogens and Global Health, 114*(2), 64–67. https://doi.org/10.1080/20477724.2020.1725339

Bialek, S., Boundy, E., Bowen, V., Chow, N., Cohn, A., & Dowling, N. (2020). CDC COVID-19 Response Team. COVID-19 Response Team. Severe outcomes among patients with coronavirus disease 2019 (COVID-19)—United States, February 12–March 16, 2020. *MMWR Morb Mortal Wkly Rep*, *69*(12), 343–346.

Brennan, G., Kitzman, J. O., Rothenburg, S., Shendure, J., & Geballe, A. P. (2014). Adaptive Gene Amplification As an Intermediate Step in the Expansion of Virus Host Range. *PLOS Pathogens*, *10*(3), e1004002. https://doi.org/10.1371/journal.ppat.1004002

Brielle, E. S., Schneidman-Duhovny, D., & Linial, M. (2020). The SARS-CoV-2 Exerts a Distinctive Strategy for Interacting with the ACE2 Human Receptor. *Viruses*, *12*(5), 497. https://doi.org/10.3390/v12050497

Buratta, S., Tancini, B., Sagini, K., Delo, F., Chiaradia, E., Urbanelli, L., & Emiliani, C. (2020). Lysosomal Exocytosis, Exosome Release and Secretory Autophagy: The Autophagic- and Endo-Lysosomal Systems Go Extracellular. *International Journal of Molecular Sciences*, *21*(7), E2576. https://doi.org/10.3390/ijms21072576

Cascella, M., Rajnik, M., Aleem, A., Dulebohn, S. C., & Di Napoli, R. (2022). Features, Evaluation, and Treatment of Coronavirus (COVID-19). In *StatPearls*. StatPearls Publishing. http://www.ncbi.nlm.nih.gov/books/NBK554776/

CDC,2021. (n.d.). Retrieved 17 January 2021, from https://www.cdc.gov/csels/dsepd/ss1978/lesson3/index.html

Chan, J. F.-W., Kok, K.-H., Zhu, Z., Chu, H., To, K. K.-W., Yuan, S., & Yuen, K.-Y. (2020). Genomic characterization of the 2019 novel human-pathogenic coronavirus isolated from a patient with atypical pneumonia after visiting Wuhan. *Emerging Microbes & Infections*, *9*(1), 221–236. https://doi.org/10.1080/22221751.2020.1719902

Chan, J. F.-W., Yuan, S., Kok, K.-H., To, K. K.-W., Chu, H., Yang, J., Xing, F., Liu, J., Yip, C. C.-Y., Poon, R. W.-S., Tsoi, H.-W., Lo, S. K.-F., Chan, K.-H., Poon, V. K.-M., Chan, W.-M., Ip, J. D., Cai, J.-P., Cheng, V. C.-C., Chen, H., … Yuen, K.-Y. (2020). A familial cluster of pneumonia associated with the 2019 novel coronavirus indicating person-to-person transmission: A study of a family cluster. *The Lancet*, *395*(10223), 514–523. https://doi.org/10.1016/S0140-6736(20)30154-9

Chen, J. (2020). Pathogenicity and transmissibility of 2019-nCoV—A quick overview and comparison with other emerging viruses. *Microbes and Infection*, *22*(2), 69–71. https://doi.org/10.1016/j.micinf.2020.01.004

Chen, L., Liu, W., Zhang, Q., Xu, K., Ye, G., Wu, W., Sun, Z., Liu, F., Wu, K., Zhong, B., Mei, Y., Zhang, W., Chen, Y., Li, Y., Shi, M., Lan, K., & Liu, Y. (2020). RNA based mNGS approach identifies a novel human coronavirus from two individual pneumonia cases in 2019 Wuhan outbreak. *Emerging Microbes & Infections*, *9*(1), 313–319. https://doi.org/10.1080/22221751.2020.1725399

Chen, N., Zhou, M., Dong, X., Qu, J., Gong, F., Han, Y., Qiu, Y., Wang, J., Liu, Y., Wei, Y., Xia, J., Yu, T., Zhang, X., & Zhang, L. (2020). Epidemiological and clinical characteristics of 99 cases of 2019 novel coronavirus pneumonia in Wuhan, China: A descriptive study. *Lancet (London, England)*, *395*(10223), 507–513. https://doi.org/10.1016/S0140-6736(20)30211-7

Chen, Y., Liu, Q., & Guo, D. (2020). Emerging coronaviruses: Genome structure, replication, and pathogenesis. *Journal of Medical Virology*, *92*(4), 418–423. https://doi.org/10.1002/jmv.25681

Chibo, D., & Birch, C. 2006. (n.d.). Analysis of human coronavirus 229E spike and nucleoprotein genes demonstrates genetic drift between chronologically distinct strains. *Journal of General Virology*, *87*(5), 1203–1208. https://doi.org/10.1099/vir.0.81662-0

Chowdhury, K. H., Chowdhury, M. R., Mahmud, S., Tareq, A. M., Hanif, N. B., Banu, N., Reza, A. S. M. A., Emran, T. B., & Simal-Gandara, J. (2021). Drug Repurposing Approach against Novel Coronavirus Disease (COVID-19) through Virtual Screening Targeting SARS-CoV-2 Main Protease. *Biology*, *10*(1), 2. https://doi.org/10.3390/biology10010002

Cohen, J. (2020). COVID-19 shot protects monkeys. *Science*, *368*(6490), 456–457. https://doi.org/10.1126/science.368.6490.456

COVAX. (n.d.). Retrieved 19 February 2021, from https://www.who.int/initiatives/act-accelerator/covax

COVID Live—Coronavirus Statistics—Worldometer. (n.d.-a). Retrieved 29 April 2022, from https://www.worldometers.info/coronavirus/

COVID-19 Map,2020. (n.d.). Johns Hopkins Coronavirus Resource Center. Retrieved 29 April 2022, from https://coronavirus.jhu.edu/map.html

Covid-19: WHO says laboratory escape theory is "extremely unlikely" after mission to China - ProQuest. (n.d.). Retrieved 29 April 2022, from https://www.proquest.com/openview/cf9e90e7693d1a71c455c3bb55746356/1?pq-origsite=gscholar&cbl=2043523

Cunningham, A. C., Goh, H. P., & Koh, D. (2020). Treatment of COVID-19: Old tricks for new challenges. *Critical Care (London, England)*, *24*(1), 91. https://doi.org/10.1186/s13054-020-2818-6

Cyranoski, D. (2020). Mystery deepens over animal source of coronavirus. *Nature*, *579*(7797), 18–20.

de Wit, E., van Doremalen, N., Falzarano, D., & Munster, V. J. (2016). SARS and MERS: Recent insights into emerging coronaviruses. *Nature Reviews. Microbiology*, *14*(8), 523–534. https://doi.org/10.1038/nrmicro.2016.81

Devaux, C. A., Rolain, J.-M., & Raoult, D. (2020). ACE2 receptor polymorphism: Susceptibility to SARS-CoV-2, hypertension, multi-organ failure, and COVID-19 disease outcome. *Journal of Microbiology, Immunology and Infection*, *53*(3), 425–435. https://doi.org/10.1016/j.jmii.2020.04.015

Dg, A., Hj, S., Mh, K., S, L., Hs, K., J, M., Bt, K., & Sj, K. (2020). Current Status of Epidemiology, Diagnosis, Therapeutics, and Vaccines for Novel Coronavirus Disease 2019 (COVID-19). *Journal of Microbiology and Biotechnology*, *30*(3). https://doi.org/10.4014/jmb.2003.03011

Diao, B., Wang, C., Tan, Y., Chen, X., Liu, Y., Ning, L., Chen, L., Li, M., Liu, Y., Wang, G., Yuan, Z., Feng, Z., Zhang, Y., Wu, Y., & Chen, Y. (2020). Reduction and Functional Exhaustion of T Cells in Patients With Coronavirus Disease 2019 (COVID-19). *Frontiers in Immunology*, *11*. https://www.frontiersin.org/article/10.3389/fimmu.2020.00827

Dong, E., Du, H., & Gardner, L. (2020). An interactive web-based dashboard to track COVID-19 in real time. *The Lancet Infectious Diseases*, *20*(5), 533–534. https://doi.org/10.1016/S1473-3099(20)30120-1

Dowd, J. B., & Aiello, A. (2009). Socioeconomic Differentials in Immune Response in the U.S. *Epidemiology (Cambridge, Mass.)*, *20*(6), 902–908. https://doi.org/10.1097/EDE.0b013e3181bb5302

Du, L., He, Y., Zhou, Y., Liu, S., Zheng, B.-J., & Jiang, S. (2009). The spike protein of SARS-CoV — a target for vaccine and therapeutic development. *Nature Reviews Microbiology*, *7*(3), 226–236. https://doi.org/10.1038/nrmicro2090

Ellinghaus, D., Degenhardt, F., Bujanda, L., Buti, M., Albillos, A., Invernizzi, P., Fernández, J., Prati, D., Baselli, G., Asselta, R., Grimsrud, M. M., Milani, C., Aziz, F., Kässens, J., May, S., Wendorff, M., Wienbrandt, L., Uellendahl-Werth, F., Zheng, T., … Karlsen, T. H. (2020). *The ABO blood group locus and a chromosome 3 gene cluster associate with SARS-CoV-2 respiratory failure in an Italian-Spanish genome-wide association analysis* (p. 2020.05.31.20114991). medRxiv. https://doi.org/10.1101/2020.05.31.20114991

Ergönül, Ö., Akyol, M., Tanrıöver, C., Tiemeier, H., Petersen, E., Petrosillo, N., & Gönen, M. (2021). National case fatality rates of the COVID-19 pandemic. *Clinical Microbiology and Infection*, *27*(1), 118–124. https://doi.org/10.1016/j.cmi.2020.09.024

Fang, Y., Zhang, H., Xie, J., Lin, M., Ying, L., Pang, P., & Ji, W. (2020). Sensitivity of Chest CT for COVID-19: Comparison to RT-PCR. *Radiology*, *296*(2), E115–E117. https://doi.org/10.1148/radiol.2020200432

Fauver, J. R., Petrone, M. E., Hodcroft, E. B., Shioda, K., Ehrlich, H. Y., Watts, A. G., Vogels, C. B. F., Brito, A. F., Alpert, T., Muyombwe, A., Razeq, J., Downing, R., Cheemarla, N. R., Wyllie, A. L., Kalinich, C. C., Ott, I. M., Quick, J., Loman, N. J., Neugebauer, K. M., … Grubaugh, N. D. (2020). Coast-to-Coast Spread of SARS-CoV-2 during the Early

Epidemic in the United States. *Cell, 181*(5), 990-996.e5. https://doi.org/10.1016/j.cell.2020.04.021

Gao, J., Tian, Z., & Yang, X. (2020). Breakthrough: Chloroquine phosphate has shown apparent efficacy in treatment of COVID-19 associated pneumonia in clinical studies. *BioScience Trends*, *advpub*, 2020.01047. https://doi.org/10.5582/bst.2020.01047

Gao, Y., Yan, L., Huang, Y., Liu, F., Zhao, Y., Cao, L., Wang, T., Sun, Q., Ming, Z., Zhang, L., Ge, J., Zheng, L., Zhang, Y., Wang, H., Zhu, Y., Zhu, C., Hu, T., Hua, T., Zhang, B., … Rao, Z. (2020a). *Structure of RNA-dependent RNA polymerase from 2019-nCoV, a major antiviral drug target* (p. 2020.03.16.993386). bioRxiv. https://doi.org/10.1101/2020.03.16.993386

Gao, Y., Yan, L., Huang, Y., Liu, F., Zhao, Y., Cao, L., Wang, T., Sun, Q., Ming, Z., Zhang, L., Ge, J., Zheng, L., Zhang, Y., Wang, H., Zhu, Y., Zhu, C., Hu, T., Hua, T., Zhang, B., … Rao, Z. (2020b). Structure of the RNA-dependent RNA polymerase from COVID-19 virus. *Science*, *368*(6492), 779–782. https://doi.org/10.1126/science.abb7498

Garg, S., Kim, L., Whitaker, M., O'Halloran, A., Cummings, C., Holstein, R., Prill, M., Chai, S. J., Kirley, P. D., Alden, N. B., Kawasaki, B., Yousey-Hindes, K., Niccolai, L., Anderson, E. J., Openo, K. P., Weigel, A., Monroe, M. L., Ryan, P., Henderson, J., … Fry, A. (2020). Hospitalization Rates and Characteristics of Patients Hospitalized with Laboratory-Confirmed Coronavirus Disease 2019—COVID-NET, 14 States, March 1–30, 2020. *Morbidity and Mortality Weekly Report*, *69*(15), 458–464. https://doi.org/10.15585/mmwr.mm6915e3

Ge, H., Wang, X., Yuan, X., Xiao, G., Wang, C., Deng, T., Yuan, Q., & Xiao, X. (2020). The epidemiology and clinical information about COVID-19. *European Journal of Clinical*

Microbiology & Infectious Diseases, *39*(6), 1011–1019. https://doi.org/10.1007/s10096-020-03874-z

Gharizadeh, B., Yue, J., Yu, M., Liu, Y., Zhou, M., Lu, D., & Zhang, J. (2021). Navigating the Pandemic Response Life Cycle: Molecular Diagnostics and Immunoassays in the Context of COVID-19 Management. *IEEE Reviews in Biomedical Engineering*, *14*, 30–47. https://doi.org/10.1109/RBME.2020.2991444

Ghinai, I., McPherson, T. D., Hunter, J. C., Kirking, H. L., Christiansen, D., Joshi, K., Rubin, R., Morales-Estrada, S., Black, S. R., Pacilli, M., Fricchione, M. J., Chugh, R. K., Walblay, K. A., Ahmed, N. S., Stoecker, W. C., Hasan, N. F., Burdsall, D. P., Reese, H. E., Wallace, M., … Uyeki, T. M. (2020). First known person-to-person transmission of severe acute respiratory syndrome coronavirus 2 (SARS-CoV-2) in the USA. *The Lancet*, *395*(10230), 1137–1144. https://doi.org/10.1016/S0140-6736(20)30607-3

Gierer, S., Bertram, S., Kaup, F., Wrensch, F., Heurich, A., Krämer-Kühl, A., Welsch, K., Winkler, M., Meyer, B., Drosten, C., Dittmer, U., von Hahn, T., Simmons, G., Hofmann, H., & Pöhlmann, S. (2013). The Spike Protein of the Emerging Betacoronavirus EMC Uses a Novel Coronavirus Receptor for Entry, Can Be Activated by TMPRSS2, and Is Targeted by Neutralizing Antibodies. *Journal of Virology*, *87*(10), 5502–5511. https://doi.org/10.1128/JVI.00128-13

GoodRx Health. (n.d.). Retrieved 16 January 2021, from https://www.goodrx.com/conditions/covid-19/coronavirus-covid-19-testing-updates-methods-cost-availability

Guan, W., Ni, Z., Hu, Y., Liang, W., Ou, C., He, J., Liu, L., Shan, H., Lei, C., Hui, D. S. C., Du, B., Li, L., Zeng, G., Yuen, K.-Y., Chen, R., Tang, C., Wang, T., Chen, P., Xiang, J., …

Zhong, N. (2020). Clinical Characteristics of Coronavirus Disease 2019 in China. *New England Journal of Medicine*, *382*(18), 1708–1720. https://doi.org/10.1056/NEJMoa2002032

Guan, Y., Zheng, B. J., He, Y. Q., Liu, X. L., Zhuang, Z. X., Cheung, C. L., Luo, S. W., Li, P. H., Zhang, L. J., Guan, Y. J., Butt, K. M., Wong, K. L., Chan, K. W., Lim, W., Shortridge, K. F., Yuen, K. Y., Peiris, J. S. M., & Poon, L. L. M. (2003). Isolation and characterization of viruses related to the SARS coronavirus from animals in southern China. *Science (New York, N.Y.)*, *302*(5643), 276–278. https://doi.org/10.1126/science.1087139

Guaraldi, G., Meschiari, M., Cozzi-Lepri, A., Milic, J., Tonelli, R., Menozzi, M., Franceschini, E., Cuomo, G., Orlando, G., Borghi, V., Santoro, A., Di Gaetano, M., Puzzolante, C., Carli, F., Bedini, A., Corradi, L., Fantini, R., Castaniere, I., Tabbì, L., … Mussini, C. (2020). Tocilizumab in patients with severe COVID-19: A retrospective cohort study. *The Lancet Rheumatology*, *2*(8), e474–e484. https://doi.org/10.1016/S2665-9913(20)30173-9

Gupte, M., Boustany-Kari, C. M., Bharadwaj, K., Police, S., Thatcher, S., Gong, M. C., English, V. L., & Cassis, L. A. (2008). ACE2 is expressed in mouse adipocytes and regulated by a high-fat diet. *American Journal of Physiology-Regulatory, Integrative and Comparative Physiology*, *295*(3), R781–R788. https://doi.org/10.1152/ajpregu.00183.2008

Hadfield, J., Megill, C., Bell, S. M., Huddleston, J., Potter, B., Callender, C., Sagulenko, P., Bedford, T., & Neher, R. A. (2018). Nextstrain: Real-time tracking of pathogen evolution. *Bioinformatics (Oxford, England)*, *34*(23), 4121–4123. https://doi.org/10.1093/bioinformatics/bty407

Hamming, I., Timens, W., Bulthuis, M., Lely, A., Navis, G., & van Goor, H. (2004). Tissue distribution of ACE2 protein, the functional receptor for SARS coronavirus. A first step in understanding SARS pathogenesis. *The Journal of Pathology*, *203*(2), 631–637. https://doi.org/10.1002/path.1570

Hanna, R., Dalvi, S., Sălăgean, T., Pop, I. D., Bordea, I. R., & Benedicenti, S. (2021). Understanding COVID-19 Pandemic: Molecular Mechanisms and Potential Therapeutic Strategies. An Evidence-Based Review. *Journal of Inflammation Research*, *14*, 13–56. https://doi.org/10.2147/JIR.S282213

Hartenian, E., Nandakumar, D., Lari, A., Ly, M., Tucker, J. M., & Glaunsinger, B. A. (2020). The molecular virology of coronaviruses. *Journal of Biological Chemistry*, *295*(37), 12910–12934. https://doi.org/10.1074/jbc.REV120.013930

Hassan, S. A., Sheikh, F. N., Jamal, S., Ezeh, J. K., & Akhtar, A. (2020). Coronavirus (COVID-19): A Review of Clinical Features, Diagnosis, and Treatment. *Cureus*, *12*(3). https://doi.org/10.7759/cureus.7355

Hawks, L., Woolhandler, S., & McCormick, D. (2020). COVID-19 in Prisons and Jails in the United States. *JAMA Internal Medicine*, *180*(8), 1041–1042. https://doi.org/10.1001/jamainternmed.2020.1856

Hoque, M. N., Chaudhury, A., Akanda, M. A. M., Hossain, M. A., & Islam, M. T. (2020). Genomic diversity and evolution, diagnosis, prevention, and therapeutics of the pandemic COVID-19 disease. *PeerJ*, *8*, e9689. https://doi.org/10.7717/peerj.9689

Hossain, M. J. (2020). Is Bangladesh Moving toward Herd Immunity? Current COVID-19 Perspective. *Bangladesh Journal of Infectious Diseases*, S63–S66. https://doi.org/10.3329/bjid.v7i00.50166

Hossain, M. J., Ahmmed, F., Kuddus, M. R., Alam, S., & Rahman, S. A. (2021). Exploring public awareness and spreading pattern analysis of COVID-19 outbreak in Bangladesh. *Bangladesh Journal of Medical Science*, 108–117. https://doi.org/10.3329/bjms.v20i5.55403

Hossain, M. J., Jannat, T., Brishty, S. R., Roy, U., Mitra, S., Rafi, M. O., Islam, M. R., Nesa, M. L., Islam, M. A., & Emran, T. B. (2021). Clinical Efficacy and Safety of Antiviral Drugs in the Extended Use against COVID-19: What We Know So Far. *Biologics*, *1*(2), 252–284. https://doi.org/10.3390/biologics1020016

Hossain, M. J., Kuddus, M. R., & Rahman, S. M. A. (2021). Knowledge, Attitudes, and Behavioral Responses Toward COVID-19 During Early Phase in Bangladesh: A Questionnaire-Based Study. *Asia-Pacific Journal of Public Health*, *33*(1), 141–144. https://doi.org/10.1177/1010539520977328

Hossain, M. J., Kuddus, M. R., Rashid, M. A., & Sultan, M. Z. (2021). Understanding and Dealing the SARS-CoV-2 Infection: An Updated Concise Review. *Bangladesh Pharmaceutical Journal*, *24*(1), 61–75. https://doi.org/10.3329/bpj.v24i1.51637

Hossain, M. J., & Rahman, S. M. A. (2021). Repurposing therapeutic agents against SARS-CoV-2 infection: Most promising and neoteric progress. *Expert Review of Anti-Infective Therapy*, *19*(8), 1009–1027. https://doi.org/10.1080/14787210.2021.1864327

Hossain, M. J., Soma, M. A., Islam, M. R., & Emran, T. B. (2021). Urgent call for actionable measures to fight the current co-epidemic of dengue burden during the SARS-CoV-2 delta variant era in South-Asia. *Ethics, Medicine, and Public Health*, *19*, 100726. https://doi.org/10.1016/j.jemep.2021.100726

Hossain, Md. J., Ahmmed, F., Rahman, S. M. A., Sanam, S., Emran, T. B., & Mitra, S. (2021). Impact of online education on fear of academic delay and psychological distress among university students following one year of COVID-19 outbreak in Bangladesh. *Heliyon, 7*(6), e07388. https://doi.org/10.1016/j.heliyon.2021.e07388

Huang, C., Wang, Y., Li, X., Ren, L., Zhao, J., Hu, Y., Zhang, L., Fan, G., Xu, J., Gu, X., Cheng, Z., Yu, T., Xia, J., Wei, Y., Wu, W., Xie, X., Yin, W., Li, H., Liu, M., … Cao, B. (2020). Clinical features of patients infected with 2019 novel coronavirus in Wuhan, China. *The Lancet, 395*(10223), 497–506. https://doi.org/10.1016/S0140-6736(20)30183-5

Hui, D. S., I Azhar, E., Madani, T. A., Ntoumi, F., Kock, R., Dar, O., Ippolito, G., Mchugh, T. D., Memish, Z. A., Drosten, C., Zumla, A., & Petersen, E. (2020). The continuing 2019-nCoV epidemic threat of novel coronaviruses to global health—The latest 2019 novel coronavirus outbreak in Wuhan, China. *International Journal of Infectious Diseases, 91*, 264–266. https://doi.org/10.1016/j.ijid.2020.01.009

Hussain, M., Jabeen, N., Amanullah, A., Baig, A. A., Aziz, B., Shabbir, S., & Raza, F. (2020). *Structural Basis of SARS-CoV-2 Spike Protein Priming by TMPRSS2* (p. 2020.04.21.052639). bioRxiv. https://doi.org/10.1101/2020.04.21.052639

Ji, W., Wang, W., Zhao, X., Zai, J., & Li, X. (2020). Cross-species transmission of the newly identified coronavirus 2019-nCoV. *Journal of Medical Virology, 92*(4), 433–440. https://doi.org/10.1002/jmv.25682

Jiang, S., Hillyer, C., & Du, L. (2020). Neutralizing Antibodies against SARS-CoV-2 and Other Human Coronaviruses. *Trends in Immunology, 41*(5), 355–359. https://doi.org/10.1016/j.it.2020.03.007

Johns Hopkins Coronavirus Resource Center. (n.d.). Johns Hopkins Coronavirus Resource Center. Retrieved 16 January 2021, from https://coronavirus.jhu.edu/testing/testing-faq

Kahn, J. S., & McIntosh, K. (2005). History and Recent Advances in Coronavirus Discovery. *The Pediatric Infectious Disease Journal*, *24*(11), S223. https://doi.org/10.1097/01.inf.0000188166.17324.60

Kakodkar, P., Kaka, N., & Baig, M. N. (2020). A Comprehensive Literature Review on the Clinical Presentation, and Management of the Pandemic Coronavirus Disease 2019 (COVID-19). *Cureus*, *12*(4). https://doi.org/10.7759/cureus.7560

Kampf, G., Todt, D., Pfaender, S., & Steinmann, E. (2020). Persistence of coronaviruses on inanimate surfaces and their inactivation with biocidal agents. *Journal of Hospital Infection*, *104*(3), 246–251. https://doi.org/10.1016/j.jhin.2020.01.022

Khadim Sheikh, H., Arshad, T., Mohammad, Z. S., Arshad, I., & Hassan, M. (2020). *Repurposed Single Inhibitor for Serine Protease and Spike Glycoproteins of SAR-CoV-*. https://doi.org/10.26434/chemrxiv.12192660.v1

Kile, G., Amanda, W., Rachel, D., Sara, G., Robert, W., Susan, M., & A. Joy, A. (n.d.). *What tests could potentially be used for the screening, diagnosis and monitoring of COVID-19 and what are their advantages and disadvantages?* The Centre for Evidence-Based Medicine. Retrieved 29 April 2022, from https://www.cebm.net/covid-19/what-tests-could-potentially-be-used-for-the-screening-diagnosis-and-monitoring-of-covid-19-and-what-are-their-advantages-and-disadvantages/

Kim, J. H., Marks, F., & Clemens, J. D. (2021). Looking beyond COVID-19 vaccine phase 3 trials. *Nature Medicine*, *27*(2), 205–211. https://doi.org/10.1038/s41591-021-01230-y

Kocher, K., Delot-Vilain, A., Spencer, D., LoTempio, J., & Délot, E. C. (2021). Paucity and Disparity of Publicly Available Sex-Disaggregated Data for the COVID-19 Epidemic Hamper Evidence-Based Decision-Making. *Archives of Sexual Behavior*, *50*(2), 407–426. https://doi.org/10.1007/s10508-020-01882-w

Kopel, J., Perisetti, A., Roghani, A., Aziz, M., Gajendran, M., & Goyal, H. (2020). Racial and Gender-Based Differences in COVID-19. *Frontiers in Public Health*, *8*. https://www.frontiersin.org/article/10.3389/fpubh.2020.00418

Korber, B., Fischer, W. M., Gnanakaran, S., Yoon, H., Theiler, J., Abfalterer, W., Hengartner, N., Giorgi, E. E., Bhattacharya, T., Foley, B., Hastie, K. M., Parker, M. D., Partridge, D. G., Evans, C. M., Freeman, T. M., de Silva, T. I., Angyal, A., Brown, R. L., Carrilero, L., … Montefiori, D. C. (2020). Tracking Changes in SARS-CoV-2 Spike: Evidence that D614G Increases Infectivity of the COVID-19 Virus. *Cell*, *182*(4), 812-827.e19. https://doi.org/10.1016/j.cell.2020.06.043

Lan, S.-H., Lai, C.-C., Huang, H.-T., Chang, S.-P., Lu, L.-C., & Hsueh, P.-R. (2020). Tocilizumab for severe COVID-19: A systematic review and meta-analysis. *International Journal of Antimicrobial Agents*, *56*(3), 106103. https://doi.org/10.1016/j.ijantimicag.2020.106103

Leung, N. H. L., Chu, D. K. W., Shiu, E. Y. C., Chan, K.-H., McDevitt, J. J., Hau, B. J. P., Yen, H.-L., Li, Y., Ip, D. K. M., Peiris, J. S. M., Seto, W.-H., Leung, G. M., Milton, D. K., & Cowling, B. J. (2020). Respiratory virus shedding in exhaled breath and efficacy of face masks. *Nature Medicine*, *26*(5), 676–680. https://doi.org/10.1038/s41591-020-0843-2

Li, F. (2016). Structure, Function, and Evolution of Coronavirus Spike Proteins. *Annual Review of Virology*, *3*(1), 237–261. https://doi.org/10.1146/annurev-virology-110615-042301

Li, R., Pei, S., Chen, B., Song, Y., Zhang, T., Yang, W., & Shaman, J. (2020). Substantial undocumented infection facilitates the rapid dissemination of novel coronavirus (SARS-CoV-2). *Science*, *368*(6490), 489–493. https://doi.org/10.1126/science.abb3221

Li, W., Shi, Z., Yu, M., Ren, W., Smith, C., Epstein, J. H., Wang, H., Crameri, G., Hu, Z., Zhang, H., Zhang, J., McEachern, J., Field, H., Daszak, P., Eaton, B. T., Zhang, S., & Wang, L.-F. (2005). Bats are natural reservoirs of SARS-like coronaviruses. *Science (New York, N.Y.)*, *310*(5748), 676–679. https://doi.org/10.1126/science.1118391

Liu, P., Chen, W., & Chen, J.-P. (2019). Viral Metagenomics Revealed Sendai Virus and Coronavirus Infection of Malayan Pangolins (Manis javanica). *Viruses*, *11*(11), 979. https://doi.org/10.3390/v11110979

Lu, G., Wang, Q., & Gao, G. F. (2015). Bat-to-human: Spike features determining 'host jump' of coronaviruses SARS-CoV, MERS-CoV, and beyond. *Trends in Microbiology*, *23*(8), 468–478. https://doi.org/10.1016/j.tim.2015.06.003

Lu, R., Zhao, X., Li, J., Niu, P., Yang, B., Wu, H., Wang, W., Song, H., Huang, B., Zhu, N., Bi, Y., Ma, X., Zhan, F., Wang, L., Hu, T., Zhou, H., Hu, Z., Zhou, W., Zhao, L., … Tan, W. (2020). Genomic characterisation and epidemiology of 2019 novel coronavirus: Implications for virus origins and receptor binding. *The Lancet*, *395*(10224), 565–574. https://doi.org/10.1016/S0140-6736(20)30251-8

Mahmud, S., Paul, G. K., Afroze, M., Islam, S., Gupt, S. B. R., Razu, M. H., Biswas, S., Zaman, S., Uddin, M. S., Khan, M., Cacciola, N. A., Emran, T. B., Saleh, M. A., Capasso, R., & Simal-Gandara, J. (2021). Efficacy of Phytochemicals Derived from Avicennia officinalis for the Management of COVID-19: A Combined In Silico and Biochemical Study. *Molecules*, *26*(8), 2210. https://doi.org/10.3390/molecules26082210

Malik, Y. A. (2020). Properties of coronavirus and SARS-CoV-2. *The Malaysian Journal of Pathology*, *42*(1), 3–11.

McCreary, E. K., Pogue, J. M., & on behalf of the Society of Infectious Diseases Pharmacists. (2020). Coronavirus Disease 2019 Treatment: A Review of Early and Emerging Options. *Open Forum Infectious Diseases*, *7*(4), ofaa105. https://doi.org/10.1093/ofid/ofaa105

Millet, J. K., & Whittaker, G. R. (2014). Host cell entry of Middle East respiratory syndrome coronavirus after two-step, furin-mediated activation of the spike protein. *Proceedings of the National Academy of Sciences*, *111*(42), 15214–15219. https://doi.org/10.1073/pnas.1407087111

Mir, J. M., & Maurya, R. C. (2021). Nitric oxide as a therapeutic option for COVID-19 treatment: A concise perspective. *New Journal of Chemistry*, *45*(4), 1774–1784. https://doi.org/10.1039/D0NJ03823G

Nainu, F., Abidin, R. S., Bahar, Muh. A., Frediansyah, A., Emran, T. B., Rabaan, A. A., Dhama, K., & Harapan, H. (2020). SARS-CoV-2 reinfection and implications for vaccine development. *Human Vaccines & Immunotherapeutics*, *16*(12), 3061–3073. https://doi.org/10.1080/21645515.2020.1830683

Nao, N., Yamagishi, J., Miyamoto, H., Igarashi, M., Manzoor, R., Ohnuma, A., Tsuda, Y., Furuyama, W., Shigeno, A., Kajihara, M., Kishida, N., Yoshida, R., & Takada, A. (2017). Genetic Predisposition To Acquire a Polybasic Cleavage Site for Highly Pathogenic Avian Influenza Virus Hemagglutinin. *MBio*, *8*(1), e02298-16. https://doi.org/10.1128/mBio.02298-16

New York Times. (n.d.). Retrieved 26 November 2020, from https://www.nytimes.com/interactive/2020/science/coronavirus-vaccine-tracker.html

Novel Coronavirus – China. (n.d.). Retrieved 29 April 2022, from https://www.who.int/emergencies/disease-outbreak-news/item/2020-DON233

Ong, S. W. X., Tan, Y. K., Chia, P. Y., Lee, T. H., Ng, O. T., Wong, M. S. Y., & Marimuthu, K. (2020). Air, Surface Environmental, and Personal Protective Equipment Contamination by Severe Acute Respiratory Syndrome Coronavirus 2 (SARS-CoV-2) From a Symptomatic Patient. *JAMA*, *323*(16), 1610–1612. https://doi.org/10.1001/jama.2020.3227

Osong Public Health and Research Perspectives 2020. (2020). *Early Epidemiological and Clinical Characteristics of 28 Cases of Coronavirus Disease in South Korea*, *11*(1), 8–14. https://doi.org/10.24171/j.phrp.2020.11.1.03

Otter, J. A., Donskey, C., Yezli, S., Douthwaite, S., Goldenberg, S. D., & Weber, D. J. (2016). Transmission of SARS and MERS coronaviruses and influenza virus in healthcare settings: The possible role of dry surface contamination. *Journal of Hospital Infection*, *92*(3), 235–250. https://doi.org/10.1016/j.jhin.2015.08.027

P, S., X, L., C, X., W, S., & B, P. (2020). Understanding of COVID-19 based on current evidence. *Journal of Medical Virology*, *92*(6). https://doi.org/10.1002/jmv.25722

P, Z., Xl, Y., Xg, W., B, H., L, Z., W, Z., Hr, S., Y, Z., B, L., Cl, H., Hd, C., J, C., Y, L., H, G., Rd, J., Mq, L., Y, C., Xr, S., X, W., … Zl, S. (2020). A pneumonia outbreak associated with a new coronavirus of probable bat origin. *Nature*, *579*(7798). https://doi.org/10.1038/s41586-020-2012-7

Paraskevis, D., Kostaki, E. G., Magiorkinis, G., Panayiotakopoulos, G., Sourvinos, G., & Tsiodras, S. (2020). Full-genome evolutionary analysis of the novel corona virus (2019-nCoV) rejects the hypothesis of emergence as a result of a recent recombination event.

Infection, Genetics and Evolution, *79*, 104212. https://doi.org/10.1016/j.meegid.2020.104212

Park, J.-E., Li, K., Barlan, A., Fehr, A. R., Perlman, S., McCray, P. B., & Gallagher, T. (2016). Proteolytic processing of Middle East respiratory syndrome coronavirus spikes expands virus tropism. *Proceedings of the National Academy of Sciences of the United States of America*, *113*(43), 12262–12267. https://doi.org/10.1073/pnas.1608147113

Paules, C. I., Marston, H. D., & Fauci, A. S. (2020). Coronavirus Infections—More Than Just the Common Cold. *JAMA*, *323*(8), 707–708. https://doi.org/10.1001/jama.2020.0757

Peiris, J. S. M., Guan, Y., & Yuen, K. Y. (2004). Severe acute respiratory syndrome. *Nature Medicine*, *10*(12 Suppl), S88-97. https://doi.org/10.1038/nm1143

Poduri, R., Joshi, G., & Jagadeesh, G. (2020). Drugs targeting various stages of the SARS-CoV-2 life cycle: Exploring promising drugs for the treatment of Covid-19. *Cellular Signalling*, *74*, 109721. https://doi.org/10.1016/j.cellsig.2020.109721

Q, L., X, G., P, W., X, W., L, Z., Y, T., R, R., Ksm, L., Ehy, L., Jy, W., X, X., N, X., Y, W., C, L., Q, C., D, L., T, L., J, Z., M, L., … Z, F. (2020). Early Transmission Dynamics in Wuhan, China, of Novel Coronavirus-Infected Pneumonia. *The New England Journal of Medicine*, *382*(13). https://doi.org/10.1056/NEJMoa2001316

Qin, P., Du, E.-Z., Luo, W.-T., Yang, Y.-L., Zhang, Y.-Q., Wang, B., & Huang, Y.-W. (2019). Characteristics of the Life Cycle of Porcine Deltacoronavirus (PDCoV) In Vitro: Replication Kinetics, Cellular Ultrastructure and Virion Morphology, and Evidence of Inducing Autophagy. *Viruses*, *11*(5), 455. https://doi.org/10.3390/v11050455

Rabaan, A. A., Al-Ahmed, S. H., Garout, M. A., Al-Qaaneh, A. M., Sule, A. A., Tirupathi, R., Mutair, A. A., Alhumaid, S., Hasan, A., Dhawan, M., Tiwari, R., Sharun, K., Mohapatra,

R. K., Mitra, S., Emran, T. B., Bilal, M., Singh, R., Alyami, S. A., Moni, M. A., & Dhama, K. (2021). Diverse Immunological Factors Influencing Pathogenesis in Patients with COVID-19: A Review on Viral Dissemination, Immunotherapeutic Options to Counter Cytokine Storm and Inflammatory Responses. *Pathogens*, *10*(5), 565. https://doi.org/10.3390/pathogens10050565

Rabaan, A. A., Al-Ahmed, S. H., Muhammad, J., Khan, A., Sule, A. A., Tirupathi, R., Mutair, A. A., Alhumaid, S., Al-Omari, A., Dhawan, M., Tiwari, R., Sharun, K., Mohapatra, R. K., Mitra, S., Bilal, M., Alyami, S. A., Emran, T. B., Moni, M. A., & Dhama, K. (2021). Role of Inflammatory Cytokines in COVID-19 Patients: A Review on Molecular Mechanisms, Immune Functions, Immunopathology and Immunomodulatory Drugs to Counter Cytokine Storm. *Vaccines*, *9*(5), 436. https://doi.org/10.3390/vaccines9050436

Rajgor, D. D., Lee, M. H., Archuleta, S., Bagdasarian, N., & Quek, S. C. (2020). The many estimates of the COVID-19 case fatality rate. *The Lancet Infectious Diseases*, *20*(7), 776–777. https://doi.org/10.1016/S1473-3099(20)30244-9

Rakib, A., Nain, Z., Sami, S. A., Mahmud, S., Islam, A., Ahmed, S., Siddiqui, A. B. F., Babu, S. M. O. F., Hossain, P., Shahriar, A., Nainu, F., Emran, T. B., & Simal-Gandara, J. (2021). A molecular modelling approach for identifying antiviral selenium-containing heterocyclic compounds that inhibit the main protease of SARS-CoV-2: An in silico investigation. *Briefings in Bioinformatics*, *22*(2), 1476–1498. https://doi.org/10.1093/bib/bbab045

Rakib, A., Sami, S. A., Islam, M. A., Ahmed, S., Faiz, F. B., Khanam, B. H., Marma, K. K. S., Rahman, M., Uddin, M. M. N., Nainu, F., Emran, T. B., & Simal-Gandara, J. (2020). Epitope-Based Immunoinformatics Approach on Nucleocapsid Protein of Severe Acute

Respiratory Syndrome-Coronavirus-2. *Molecules*, *25*(21), 5088. https://doi.org/10.3390/molecules25215088

Ramanathan, A., Robb, G. B., & Chan, S.-H. (2016). mRNA capping: Biological functions and applications. *Nucleic Acids Research*, *44*(16), 7511–7526. https://doi.org/10.1093/nar/gkw551

Rc, B. (2020). Covid-19 treatment update: Follow the scientific evidence. *Journal of Thrombosis and Thrombolysis*, *50*(1). https://doi.org/10.1007/s11239-020-02120-9

Ren, L., Zhang, Y., Li, J., Xiao, Y., Zhang, J., Wang, Y., Chen, L., Paranhos-Baccalà, G., & Wang, J. (2015). Genetic drift of human coronavirus OC43 spike gene during adaptive evolution. *Scientific Reports*, *5*, 11451. https://doi.org/10.1038/srep11451

Romano, M., Ruggiero, A., Squeglia, F., Maga, G., & Berisio, R. (2020). A Structural View of SARS-CoV-2 RNA Replication Machinery: RNA Synthesis, Proofreading and Final Capping. *Cells*, *9*(5), E1267. https://doi.org/10.3390/cells9051267

Rosa, S. G. V., & Santos, W. C. (2020). Clinical trials on drug repositioning for COVID-19 treatment. *Revista Panamericana De Salud Publica = Pan American Journal of Public Health*, *44*, e40. https://doi.org/10.26633/RPSP.2020.40

S, P., & J, N. (2009). Coronaviruses post-SARS: Update on replication and pathogenesis. *Nature Reviews. Microbiology*, *7*(6). https://doi.org/10.1038/nrmicro2147

Samadizadeh, S., Masoudi, M., Rastegar, M., Salimi, V., Shahbaz, M. B., & Tahamtan, A. (2021). COVID-19: Why does disease severity vary among individuals? *Respiratory Medicine*, *180*, 106356. https://doi.org/10.1016/j.rmed.2021.106356

Scagnolari, C., Vicenzi, E., Bellomi, F., Stillitano, M. G., Pinna, D., Poli, G., Clementi, M., Dianzani, F., & Antonelli, G. (2004). Increased Sensitivity of Sars-Coronavirus to a

Combination of Human Type I and Type II Interferons. *Antiviral Therapy*, *9*(6), 1003–1011. https://doi.org/10.1177/135965350400900618

Sefren Geiner, T., Fatimawali, F., Nurdjannah Jane, N., Yunus, E., Rinaldi, I., Ahmad Akroman, A., Ahmed, R., Talha Bin, E., & Trina Ekawati, T. (2020). The potential of leaf extract of Pangium edule Reinw as HIV-1 protease inhibitor: A computational biology approach. *Journal of Applied Pharmaceutical Science*. https://doi.org/10.7324/JAPS.2021.110112

Seto, W., Tsang, D., Yung, R., Ching, T., Ng, T., Ho, M., Ho, L., & Peiris, J. (2003). Effectiveness of precautions against droplets and contact in prevention of nosocomial transmission of severe acute respiratory syndrome (SARS). *The Lancet*, *361*(9368), 1519–1520. https://doi.org/10.1016/S0140-6736(03)13168-6

Sevajol, M., Subissi, L., Decroly, E., Canard, B., & Imbert, I. (2014). Insights into RNA synthesis, capping, and proofreading mechanisms of SARS-coronavirus. *Virus Research*, *194*, 90–99. https://doi.org/10.1016/j.virusres.2014.10.008

Severe Acute Respiratory Syndrome (SARS). (n.d.). Retrieved 20 February 2021, from https://www.who.int/westernpacific/health-topics/severe-acute-respiratory-syndrome

Shannon, A., Le, N. T.-T., Selisko, B., Eydoux, C., Alvarez, K., Guillemot, J.-C., Decroly, E., Peersen, O., Ferron, F., & Canard, B. (2020). Remdesivir and SARS-CoV-2: Structural requirements at both nsp12 RdRp and nsp14 Exonuclease active-sites. *Antiviral Research*, *178*, 104793. https://doi.org/10.1016/j.antiviral.2020.104793

Shen, K., Yang, Y., Wang, T., Zhao, D., Jiang, Y., Jin, R., Zheng, Y., Xu, B., Xie, Z., Lin, L., Shang, Y., Lu, X., Shu, S., Bai, Y., Deng, J., Lu, M., Ye, L., Wang, X., Wang, Y., … Global Pediatric Pulmonology Alliance. (2020). Diagnosis, treatment, and prevention of

2019 novel coronavirus infection in children: Experts' consensus statement. *World Journal of Pediatrics*, *16*(3), 223–231. https://doi.org/10.1007/s12519-020-00343-7

Shereen, M. A., Khan, S., Kazmi, A., Bashir, N., & Siddique, R. (2020). COVID-19 infection: Emergence, transmission, and characteristics of human coronaviruses. *Journal of Advanced Research*, *24*, 91–98. https://doi.org/10.1016/j.jare.2020.03.005

Shormin, M., & Yusuf, M. A. (2020). Laboratory Detection of Covid19 Cases: A Systematic Review. *Bangladesh Journal of Infectious Diseases*, S11–S17. https://doi.org/10.3329/bjid.v7i0.46796

Shu, T., Huang, M., Wu, D., Ren, Y., Zhang, X., Han, Y., Mu, J., Wang, R., Qiu, Y., Zhang, D.-Y., & Zhou, X. (2020). SARS-Coronavirus-2 Nsp13 Possesses NTPase and RNA Helicase Activities That Can Be Inhibited by Bismuth Salts. *Virologica Sinica*, *35*(3), 321–329. https://doi.org/10.1007/s12250-020-00242-1

Smith, E. C., Blanc, H., Vignuzzi, M., & Denison, M. R. (2013). Coronaviruses Lacking Exoribonuclease Activity Are Susceptible to Lethal Mutagenesis: Evidence for Proofreading and Potential Therapeutics. *PLOS Pathogens*, *9*(8), e1003565. https://doi.org/10.1371/journal.ppat.1003565

Smits, S. L., Lang, A. de, Brand, J. M. A. van den, Leijten, L. M., IJcken, W. F. van, Eijkemans, M. J. C., Amerongen, G. van, Kuiken, T., Andeweg, A. C., Osterhaus, A. D. M. E., & Haagmans, B. L. (2010). Exacerbated Innate Host Response to SARS-CoV in Aged Non-Human Primates. *PLOS Pathogens*, *6*(2), e1000756. https://doi.org/10.1371/journal.ppat.1000756

Song, H.-D., Tu, C.-C., Zhang, G.-W., Wang, S.-Y., Zheng, K., Lei, L.-C., Chen, Q.-X., Gao, Y.-W., Zhou, H.-Q., Xiang, H., Zheng, H.-J., Chern, S.-W. W., Cheng, F., Pan, C.-M., Xuan,

H., Chen, S.-J., Luo, H.-M., Zhou, D.-H., Liu, Y.-F., … Zhao, G.-P. (2005). Cross-host evolution of severe acute respiratory syndrome coronavirus in palm civet and human. *Proceedings of the National Academy of Sciences*, *102*(7), 2430–2435. https://doi.org/10.1073/pnas.0409608102

Steptoe, A., Shamaei-Tousi, A., Gylfe, A., Henderson, B., Bergström, S., & Marmot, M. (2007). Socioeconomic status, pathogen burden and cardiovascular disease risk. *Heart (British Cardiac Society)*, *93*(12), 1567–1570. https://doi.org/10.1136/hrt.2006.113993

Stockman, L. J., Bellamy, R., & Garner, P. (2006). SARS: Systematic review of treatment effects. *PLoS Medicine*, *3*(9), e343. https://doi.org/10.1371/journal.pmed.0030343

Su, Z., Wen, J., McDonnell, D., Goh, E., Li, X., Šegalo, S., Ahmad, J., Cheshmehzangi, A., & Xiang, Y.-T. (2021). Vaccines are not yet a silver bullet: The imperative of continued communication about the importance of COVID-19 safety measures. *Brain, Behavior, & Immunity - Health*, *12*, 100204. https://doi.org/10.1016/j.bbih.2021.100204

Sui, J., Aird, D. R., Tamin, A., Murakami, A., Yan, M., Yammanuru, A., Jing, H., Kan, B., Liu, X., Zhu, Q., Yuan, Q.-A., Adams, G. P., Bellini, W. J., Xu, J., Anderson, L. J., & Marasco, W. A. (2008). Broadening of neutralization activity to directly block a dominant antibody-driven SARS-coronavirus evolution pathway. *PLoS Pathogens*, *4*(11), e1000197. https://doi.org/10.1371/journal.ppat.1000197

Tang, X.-C., Agnihothram, S. S., Jiao, Y., Stanhope, J., Graham, R. L., Peterson, E. C., Avnir, Y., Tallarico, A. S. C., Sheehan, J., Zhu, Q., Baric, R. S., & Marasco, W. A. (2014). Identification of human neutralizing antibodies against MERS-CoV and their role in virus adaptive evolution. *Proceedings of the National Academy of Sciences of the United States of America*, *111*(19), E2018-2026. https://doi.org/10.1073/pnas.1402074111

Tang, Z., Zhang, X., Shu, Y., Guo, M., Zhang, H., & Tao, W. (2021). Insights from nanotechnology in COVID-19 treatment. *Nano Today*, *36*, 101019. https://doi.org/10.1016/j.nantod.2020.101019

Tillu, G., Chaturvedi, S., Chopra, A., & Patwardhan, B. (2020). Public Health Approach of Ayurveda and Yoga for COVID-19 Prophylaxis. *Journal of Alternative and Complementary Medicine (New York, N.Y.)*, *26*(5), 360–364. https://doi.org/10.1089/acm.2020.0129

Tong, T., Wu, Y.-Q., Ni, W.-J., Shen, A.-Z., & Liu, S. (2020). The potential insights of Traditional Chinese Medicine on treatment of COVID-19. *Chinese Medicine*, *15*(1), 51. https://doi.org/10.1186/s13020-020-00326-w

Toniati, P., Piva, S., Cattalini, M., Garrafa, E., Regola, F., Castelli, F., Franceschini, F., Airò, P., Bazzani, C., Beindorf, E.-A., Berlendis, M., Bezzi, M., Bossini, N., Castellano, M., Cattaneo, S., Cavazzana, I., Contessi, G.-B., Crippa, M., Delbarba, A., … Latronico, N. (2020). Tocilizumab for the treatment of severe COVID-19 pneumonia with hyperinflammatory syndrome and acute respiratory failure: A single center study of 100 patients in Brescia, Italy. *Autoimmunity Reviews*, *19*(7), 102568. https://doi.org/10.1016/j.autrev.2020.102568

Totura, A. L., & Baric, R. S. (2012). SARS coronavirus pathogenesis: Host innate immune responses and viral antagonism of interferon. *Current Opinion in Virology*, *2*(3), 264–275. https://doi.org/10.1016/j.coviro.2012.04.004

Turner, A. J., Hiscox, J. A., & Hooper, N. M. (2004). ACE2: From vasopeptidase to SARS virus receptor. *Trends in Pharmacological Sciences*, *25*(6), 291–294. https://doi.org/10.1016/j.tips.2004.04.001

Uddin, M., Mustafa, F., Rizvi, T. A., Loney, T., Al Suwaidi, H., Al-Marzouqi, A. H. H., Kamal Eldin, A., Alsabeeha, N., Adrian, T. E., Stefanini, C., Nowotny, N., Alsheikh-Ali, A., & Senok, A. C. (2020). SARS-CoV-2/COVID-19: Viral Genomics, Epidemiology, Vaccines, and Therapeutic Interventions. *Viruses*, *12*(5), 526. https://doi.org/10.3390/v12050526

Uras, U. (n.d.). *Coronavirus: Comparing COVID-19, SARS and MERS*. Retrieved 16 January 2021, from https://www.aljazeera.com/news/2020/4/8/coronavirus-comparing-covid-19-sars-and-mers

van Doremalen, N., Bushmaker, T., Morris, D. H., Holbrook, M. G., Gamble, A., Williamson, B. N., Tamin, A., Harcourt, J. L., Thornburg, N. J., Gerber, S. I., Lloyd-Smith, J. O., de Wit, E., & Munster, V. J. (2020). Aerosol and Surface Stability of SARS-CoV-2 as Compared with SARS-CoV-1. *The New England Journal of Medicine*, *382*(16), 1564–1567. https://doi.org/10.1056/NEJMc2004973

Vijgen, L., Keyaerts, E., Lemey, P., Moës, E., Li, S., Vandamme, A.-M., & Van Ranst, M. (2005). Circulation of genetically distinct contemporary human coronavirus OC43 strains. *Virology*, *337*(1), 85–92. https://doi.org/10.1016/j.virol.2005.04.010

Wan, Y., Shang, J., Graham, R., Baric, R. S., & Li, F. (n.d.). Receptor Recognition by the Novel Coronavirus from Wuhan: An Analysis Based on Decade-Long Structural Studies of SARS Coronavirus. *Journal of Virology*, *94*(7), e00127-20. https://doi.org/10.1128/JVI.00127-20

Wang, W., Tang, J., & Wei, F. (2020). Updated understanding of the outbreak of 2019 novel coronavirus (2019-nCoV) in Wuhan, China. *Journal of Medical Virology*, *92*(4), 441–447. https://doi.org/10.1002/jmv.25689

Wenham, C., Smith, J., & Morgan, R. (2020). COVID-19: The gendered impacts of the outbreak. *The Lancet*, *395*(10227), 846–848. https://doi.org/10.1016/S0140-6736(20)30526-2

West, R., Kobokovich, A., Connell, N., & Gronvall, G. K. (2021). COVID-19 Antibody Tests: A Valuable Public Health Tool with Limited Relevance to Individuals. *Trends in Microbiology*, *29*(3), 214–223. https://doi.org/10.1016/j.tim.2020.11.002

WHO. (2020a). *Clinical management of severe acute respiratory infection when novel coronavirus (nCoV) infection is suspected, Interim guidance, 13 March 2020.*

WHO. (2020b). Infection prevention and control during health care when novel coronavirus (nCoV) infection is suspected. *WHO Reference Number: WHO/2019-NCoV/IPC/2020.2013. Available At.*

WHO, 2020. (n.d.). Retrieved 29 April 2022, from https://www.who.int/director-general/speeches/detail/who-director-general-s-opening-remarks-at-the-media-briefing-on-covid-19---11-may-2020

WHO,2021. (n.d.-a). Estimating Mortality from COVID-19. Retrieved 13 February 2021, from https://www.who.int/news-room/commentaries/detail/estimating-mortality-from-covid-19

WHO,2021. (n.d.-b). Advice for the Public on COVID-19. Retrieved 16 February 2021, from https://www.who.int/emergencies/diseases/novel-coronavirus-2019/advice-for-public

WONG, C. K., LAM, C. W. K., WU, A. K. L., IP, W. K., LEE, N. L. S., CHAN, I. H. S., LIT, L. C. W., HUI, D. S. C., CHAN, M. H. M., CHUNG, S. S. C., & SUNG, J. J. Y. (2004). Plasma inflammatory cytokines and chemokines in severe acute respiratory syndrome. *Clinical and Experimental Immunology*, *136*(1), 95–103. https://doi.org/10.1111/j.1365-2249.2004.02415.x

World Health Organization. (2020). *Home care for patients with suspected novel coronavirus (nCoV) infection presenting with mild symptoms and management of contacts: Interim guidance, 20 January 2020.*

Worldometer,2021. (n.d.-b). Worldometer. Retrieved 19 January 2021, from https://www.worldometers.info/coronavirus/

Wrapp, D., Wang, N., Corbett, K. S., Goldsmith, J. A., Hsieh, C.-L., Abiona, O., Graham, B. S., & McLellan, J. S. (2020). Cryo-EM structure of the 2019-nCoV spike in the prefusion conformation. *Science*, *367*(6483), 1260–1263. https://doi.org/10.1126/science.abb2507

Wu, F., Zhao, S., Yu, B., Chen, Y.-M., Wang, W., Song, Z.-G., Hu, Y., Tao, Z.-W., Tian, J.-H., Pei, Y.-Y., Yuan, M.-L., Zhang, Y.-L., Dai, F.-H., Liu, Y., Wang, Q.-M., Zheng, J.-J., Xu, L., Holmes, E. C., & Zhang, Y.-Z. (2020). A new coronavirus associated with human respiratory disease in China. *Nature*, *579*(7798), 265–269. https://doi.org/10.1038/s41586-020-2008-3

Wu, J. T., Leung, K., & Leung, G. M. (2020). Nowcasting and forecasting the potential domestic and international spread of the 2019-nCoV outbreak originating in Wuhan, China: A modelling study. *The Lancet*, *395*(10225), 689–697. https://doi.org/10.1016/S0140-6736(20)30260-9

Wu, P., Hao, X., Lau, E. H. Y., Wong, J. Y., Leung, K. S. M., Wu, J. T., Cowling, B. J., & Leung, G. M. (2020). Real-time tentative assessment of the epidemiological characteristics of novel coronavirus infections in Wuhan, China, as at 22 January 2020. *Eurosurveillance*, *25*(3), 2000044. https://doi.org/10.2807/1560-7917.ES.2020.25.3.2000044

Xu, J., Zhao, S., Teng, T., Abdalla, A. E., Zhu, W., Xie, L., Wang, Y., & Guo, X. (2020). Systematic Comparison of Two Animal-to-Human Transmitted Human Coronaviruses: SARS-CoV-2 and SARS-CoV. *Viruses*, *12*(2), 244. https://doi.org/10.3390/v12020244

Xu, X.-W., Wu, X.-X., Jiang, X.-G., Xu, K.-J., Ying, L.-J., Ma, C.-L., Li, S.-B., Wang, H.-Y., Zhang, S., Gao, H.-N., Sheng, J.-F., Cai, H.-L., Qiu, Y.-Q., & Li, L.-J. (2020). Clinical findings in a group of patients infected with the 2019 novel coronavirus (SARS-Cov-2) outside of Wuhan, China: Retrospective case series. *BMJ (Clinical Research Ed.)*, *368*, m606. https://doi.org/10.1136/bmj.m606

Xu, Z., Shi, L., Wang, Y., Zhang, J., Huang, L., Zhang, C., Liu, S., Zhao, P., Liu, H., Zhu, L., Tai, Y., Bai, C., Gao, T., Song, J., Xia, P., Dong, J., Zhao, J., & Wang, F.-S. (2020). Pathological findings of COVID-19 associated with acute respiratory distress syndrome. *The Lancet Respiratory Medicine*, *8*(4), 420–422. https://doi.org/10.1016/S2213-2600(20)30076-X

Yan, R., Zhang, Y., Li, Y., Xia, L., Guo, Y., & Zhou, Q. (2020). Structural basis for the recognition of SARS-CoV-2 by full-length human ACE2. *Science (New York, N.Y.)*, *367*(6485), 1444–1448. https://doi.org/10.1126/science.abb2762

Yang, X., Yu, Y., Xu, J., Shu, H., Xia, J., Liu, H., Wu, Y., Zhang, L., Yu, Z., Fang, M., Yu, T., Wang, Y., Pan, S., Zou, X., Yuan, S., & Shang, Y. (2020). Clinical course and outcomes of critically ill patients with SARS-CoV-2 pneumonia in Wuhan, China: A single-centered, retrospective, observational study. *The Lancet Respiratory Medicine*, *8*(5), 475–481. https://doi.org/10.1016/S2213-2600(20)30079-5

Yin, W., Mao, C., Luan, X., Shen, D.-D., Shen, Q., Su, H., Wang, X., Zhou, F., Zhao, W., Gao, M., Chang, S., Xie, Y.-C., Tian, G., Jiang, H.-W., Tao, S.-C., Shen, J., Jiang, Y., Jiang,

H., Xu, Y., … Xu, H. E. (2020). Structural basis for inhibition of the RNA-dependent RNA polymerase from SARS-CoV-2 by remdesivir. *Science (New York, N.y.)*, *368*(6498), 1499–1504. https://doi.org/10.1126/science.abc1560

Young, B., Tan, T. T., & Leo, Y. S. (2021). The place for remdesivir in COVID-19 treatment. *The Lancet Infectious Diseases*, *21*(1), 20–21. https://doi.org/10.1016/S1473-3099(20)30911-7

Yu, J., Tostanoski, L. H., Peter, L., Mercado, N. B., McMahan, K., Mahrokhian, S. H., Nkolola, J. P., Liu, J., Li, Z., Chandrashekar, A., Martinez, D. R., Loos, C., Atyeo, C., Fischinger, S., Burke, J. S., Slein, M. D., Chen, Y., Zuiani, A., Lelis, F. J. N., … Barouch, D. H. (2020). DNA vaccine protection against SARS-CoV-2 in rhesus macaques. *Science*, *369*(6505), 806–811. https://doi.org/10.1126/science.abc6284

Z, Q., C, J., H, X., Z, H., H, J., F, L., L, K., & Z, J. (2004). The life cycle of SARS coronavirus in Vero E6 cells. *Journal of Medical Virology*, *73*(3). https://doi.org/10.1002/jmv.20095

Zahedipour, F., Hosseini, S. A., Sathyapalan, T., Majeed, M., Jamialahmadi, T., Al-Rasadi, K., Banach, M., & Sahebkar, A. (2020). Potential effects of curcumin in the treatment of COVID-19 infection. *Phytotherapy Research*, *34*(11), 2911–2920. https://doi.org/10.1002/ptr.6738

Zaki, A. M., van Boheemen, S., Bestebroer, T. M., Osterhaus, A. D. M. E., & Fouchier, R. A. M. (2012). Isolation of a Novel Coronavirus from a Man with Pneumonia in Saudi Arabia. *New England Journal of Medicine*, *367*(19), 1814–1820. https://doi.org/10.1056/NEJMoa1211721

Zhang, J., Dong, X., Cao, Y., Yuan, Y., Yang, Y., Yan, Y., Akdis, C. A., & Gao, Y. (2020). Clinical characteristics of 140 patients infected with SARS-CoV-2 in Wuhan, China. *Allergy*, *75*(7), 1730–1741. https://doi.org/10.1111/all.14238

Zhang, L., Jackson, C. B., Mou, H., Ojha, A., Rangarajan, E. S., Izard, T., Farzan, M., & Choe, H. (2020). *The D614G mutation in the SARS-CoV-2 spike protein reduces S1 shedding and increases infectivity* (p. 2020.06.12.148726). bioRxiv. https://doi.org/10.1101/2020.06.12.148726

Zhang, L., Lin, D., Sun, X., Curth, U., Drosten, C., Sauerhering, L., Becker, S., Rox, K., & Hilgenfeld, R. (2020). Crystal structure of SARS-CoV-2 main protease provides a basis for design of improved α-ketoamide inhibitors. *Science*, *368*(6489), 409–412. https://doi.org/10.1126/science.abb3405

Zhang, R., Wang, X., Ni, L., Di, X., Ma, B., Niu, S., Liu, C., & Reiter, R. J. (2020). COVID-19: Melatonin as a potential adjuvant treatment. *Life Sciences*, *250*, 117583. https://doi.org/10.1016/j.lfs.2020.117583

Zhang, T., Wu, Q., & Zhang, Z. (2020). Probable Pangolin Origin of SARS-CoV-2 Associated with the COVID-19 Outbreak. *Current Biology*, *30*(7), 1346-1351.e2. https://doi.org/10.1016/j.cub.2020.03.022

Zhao, J., Yang, Y., Huang, H., Li, D., Gu, D., Lu, X., Zhang, Z., Liu, L., Liu, T., Liu, Y., He, Y., Sun, B., Wei, M., Yang, G., Wang, X., Zhang, L., Zhou, X., Xing, M., & Wang, P. G. (2021). Relationship Between the ABO Blood Group and the Coronavirus Disease 2019 (COVID-19) Susceptibility. *Clinical Infectious Diseases: An Official Publication of the Infectious Diseases Society of America*, *73*(2), 328–331. https://doi.org/10.1093/cid/ciaa1150

Zietz, M., Zucker, J., & Tatonetti, N. P. (2020). Associations between blood type and COVID-19 infection, intubation, and death. *Nature Communications*, *11*(1), 5761. https://doi.org/10.1038/s41467-020-19623-x

Zumla, A., Hui, D. S., & Perlman, S. (2015). Middle East respiratory syndrome. *The Lancet*, *386*(9997), 995–1007. https://doi.org/10.1016/S0140-6736(15)60454-8

Publisher: Eliva Press Global Ltd

Email: info@elivapress.com

Made in United States
Orlando, FL
04 November 2026

90201123R00049